Contributors

Audrey Knippa, MS, MPH, RN, CNE
Nursing Education Coordinator and
  Content Project Leader

Sheryl Sommer, PhD, MSN, RN
Director, Nursing Curriculum and
  Education Services

Brenda Ball, MEd, BSN, RN
Nursing Education Specialist

Lois Churchill, MN, RN
Nursing Education Specialist

Carrie B. Elkins, DHSc, MSN, PHCNS, BC
Nursing Education Specialist

Mary Jane Janowski, MA, BSN, RN
Nursing Resource Specialist

Karin Roberts, PhD, MSN, RN, CNE
Nursing Education Coordinator

Mendy G. Wright, DNP, MSN, RN
Nursing Education Specialist

Derek Prater, MS Journalism
Lead Product Developer and Editorial Project Leader

Erika A. Archer, BS Education, Foreign Language
Product Developer

Johanna Barnes, BA Journalism
Product Developer

Chris Crawford, BS Journalism
Product Developer

Hilary E. Groninger, BS Journalism
Product Developer

Megan E. Herre, BS Journalism
Product Developer

Amanda Lehman, BA English
Product Developer

Joanna Shindler, BA Journalism
Product Developer

Brant L. Stacy, BS Journalism, BA English
Product Developer

Consultants

Christina D. Brazier, MSN, RN

INTELLECTUAL PROPERTY NOTICE

IMPORTANT NOTICE TO THE READER

USER'S GUIDE

Welcome to the Assessment Technologies Institute® RN Community Health Nursing Review Module Edition 5.0. The mission of ATI's Content Mastery Series® review modules is to provide user-friendly compendiums of nursing knowledge that will:

- Help you locate important information quickly.

- Assist in your remediation efforts.

- Provide exercises for applying your nursing knowledge.

- Facilitate your entry into the nursing profession as a newly licensed RN.

Organization

Chapters in this review module use a nursing concepts organizing framework, beginning with an overview describing the central concept and its relevance to nursing. Subordinate themes are covered in outline form to demonstrate relationships and present the information in a clear, succinct manner. Some chapters have sections that group related concepts and contain their own overviews. These sections are included in the table of contents.

Application Exercises

Questions are provided at the end of each chapter so you can practice applying your knowledge. The Application Exercises include both NCLEX-style questions, such as multiple-choice and multiple-select items, and questions that ask you to apply your knowledge in other formats, such as short-answer and matching items. After the Application Exercises, an answer key is provided, along with rationales for the answers.

NCLEX® Connections

To prepare for the NCLEX-RN, it is important for you to understand how the content in this review module is connected to the NCLEX-RN test plan. You can find information on the detailed test plan at the National Council of State Boards of Nursing's Web site: https://www.ncsbn.org/. When reviewing content in this review module, regularly ask yourself, "How does this content fit into the test plan, and what types of questions related to this content should I expect?"

To help you in this process, we've included NCLEX Connections at the beginning of each chapter and with each question in the Application Exercises Answer Keys. The NCLEX Connections at the beginning of each chapter will point out areas of the detailed test plan that relate to the content within that chapter. The NCLEX Connections attached to the Application Exercises Answer Keys will demonstrate how each exercise fits within the detailed content outline.

These NCLEX Connections will help you understand how the detailed content outline is organized, starting with major client needs categories and subcategories and followed by related content areas and tasks. The major client needs categories are:

- Safe and Effective Care Environment

  ○ Management of Care

  ○ Safety and Infection Control

- Health Promotion and Maintenance

- Psychosocial Integrity

- Physiological Integrity
  - Basic Care and Comfort
  - Pharmacological and Parenteral Therapies
  - Reduction of Risk Potential
  - Physiological Adaptation

An NCLEX Connection might, for example, alert you that content within a chapter is related to:

- Safety and Infection Control
  - Home Safety
    - Assess need for client home modifications.

Icons

Icons are used throughout the review module to draw your attention to particular areas. Keep an eye out for these icons:

 This icon indicates an Overview, or introduction, to a particular subject matter. Descriptions and categories will typically be found in an Overview.

 This icon is used for the Application Exercises and the Application Exercises Answer Keys.

 This icon is used for NCLEX connections.

 This icon is used for gerontological content. When you see this icon, take note of information that is specific to aging or the care of older adult clients.

 This icon is used for content related to safety. When you see this icon, take note of safety concerns or steps that nurses can take to ensure client safety and a safe environment.

 This icon indicates that a media supplement, such as a graphic, an animation, or a video, is available. If you have an electronic copy of the review module, this icon will appear alongside clickable links to media supplements. If you have a hardcopy version of the review module, visit www.atitesting.com for details on how to access these features.

Feedback

ATI welcomes feedback regarding this review module. Please provide comments to: comments@ atitesting.com.

Table of Contents

Chapter 7   Continuity of Care

CHAPTER 1: OVERVIEW OF COMMUNITY HEALTH NURSING

- Foundations of Community Health Nursing

- Principles of Community Health Nursing

- Health Promotion and Disease Prevention

NCLEX® CONNECTIONS

When reviewing the content in this chapter, keep in mind the relevant sections of the NCLEX® outline, in particular:

**CLIENT NEEDS:
MANAGEMENT OF CARE**

Relevant topics/tasks include:
- Advocacy
  - Utilize advocacy resources appropriately.
- Ethical Practice
  - Practice in a manner consistent with the code of ethics for registered nurses.

**CLIENT NEEDS:
HEALTH PROMOTION AND MAINTENANCE**

Relevant topics/tasks include:
- Health and Wellness
  - Assess client perception of health status.
- Health Promotion/Disease Prevention
  - Assess and teach the client about health risks based on known population or community characteristics.
- Health Screening
  - Perform a targeted screening examination.
- Principles of Teaching/Learning
  - Select appropriate teaching methods.

Chapter 1	Overview of Community Health Nursing

Overview

- Community health nursing is a broad field of nursing that allows nurses to practice in a wide variety of settings.

- Nurses have the opportunity to promote the health and welfare of clients across the lifespan and from diverse populations.

- Nurses working in the community should have an understanding of:

  o The foundations of community health nursing

  o The principles of community health nursing

  o Health promotion and disease prevention

FOUNDATIONS OF COMMUNITY HEALTH NURSING

Overview

- Fundamental to the understanding of community health nursing is the knowledge of the history of nursing care in the community.

- Various theories and specific definitions of care guide nursing practice in the community.

History of Community Health Nursing

- Nursing care to groups of people has long been a community practice. This care to varied size groups has connections back to ancient times. While this type of health care started in a very early period and health practices have changed, the correlation to ancient practices can still be seen and has provided the basis by which community health nursing developed. Community health nursing has significance through the colonial periods, 19th century, and current times.

- Community health nursing has a nursing focus but is driven by the variety of factors affecting groups of individuals. Factors such as economic, political, and social issues impact the care delivered by the community health nurse.

TIME PERIOD	KEY PEOPLE/PLACE	FOCUS
Middle Ages	Religious Orders	Religious orders cared for disadvantaged people affected by unsanitary conditions, such as the poor or orphaned.

TIME PERIOD	KEY PEOPLE/PLACE	FOCUS
1601	English Government	The Elizabethan Poor Law was established. This law assisted the poor and disabled with receiving care.
1617	Saint Vincent de Paul	He organized a group that provided care to the ill and infirmed.
1789	Baltimore Government	The Baltimore government formed its Health Department.
1798	Act by Congress	Congress established the Marine Hospital. This facility later became the Public Health Service.
1812	Sisters of Mercy	Nuns cared for the disadvantaged.
1851	Florence Nightingale	Nightingale trained as a nurse in Germany.
1855	New Orleans	The city established a department to quarantine individuals with infectious diseases. This prompted the United States government to take a look at the tuberculosis epidemic.
1860	Florence Nightingale	Nightingale established a training school for nurses.
1864	Clara Barton	Barton established The Red Cross.
1893	Lillian Wald	Wald established the Henry Street Settlement
1925	Mary Breckinridge	Breckinridge established the Frontier Nursing Service.

Organized Health Care Beginnings

- As individuals arrived in America from Europe, so did disease. A concern for the health of settlers prompted the development of health departments that kept records and statistics on people seeking disease treatment. Based on those statistics, environmental work was instituted to control devastating illnesses and improve health. No formal hospitals existed until the development of a facility in Philadelphia.

- In 1850, a milestone took place. The Shattuck Report, developed by the Massachusetts Sanitary Commission, recommended changes to the health system. Those changes, such as control of communicable diseases, alcohol, and the teaching of preventative health care, changed the face of public health.

- Florence Nightingale is credited with the development of formal nursing care. Prior to her interest in public health, early colonial settlers followed the laws of England and established areas to care for the ill. During the Crimean War, Nightingale cared for soldiers who were dying not only from their injuries but also from disease. Nightingale's work decreased the mortality rate of soldiers by more than 30%. After the war, she returned to her home in England and formally trained nurses to care for the sick. In 1879, the United States opened the first nursing school based on Nightingale's model. Graduates held administrative positions or worked in private duty. Community health nursing developed as a result of illness of those who could not pay for private-duty nursing care.

- Visiting nurses were able to assess living conditions and suggest improvements to health care. Settlements were established. In the 1890s, Lillian Wald established the Henry Street Settlement. Wald was a progressive thinker whose work changed the face of community health. She went on to become the president of the National Organization for Public Health Nursing.

- Several monumental events occurred in the 20th century related to public health.

  o The Sheppard-Towner Act changed the course of maternal newborn care. However, this program ended in a few short years.

  o In the 1920s, Mary Breckinridge opened the Frontier Nursing Service, which is still in existence in Kentucky. Traveling to the homes of individuals in the mountainous areas of Kentucky was difficult, so nurses rode on horseback into remote areas to care for the ill.

  o Midwifery also was developed at Frontier, and the maternal newborn care to Leslie County, KY, dramatically improved because of Mary Breckinridge.

- Over the course of the 20th century, the Social Security Act was implemented, schools of nursing included course content on community/public health, and the Rural Health Clinic Services Act dictated how community health services were taught and implemented.

Community Health Nursing Theories

- Nursing theory provides the basis for our care of the community and family. Theorists have developed sound principles to guide nurses in providing quality care. Community health nursing theories include:

THEORY	DESCRIPTIONS
Nightingale's Theory of Environment	Nursing, health, and environment have a correlation in the health and illness of an individual or community.
Orem Self Care Deficit	Individuals must take actions to maintain life and health. Those actions can be performed by the individual with guidance or by a caregiver. Environmental assessment is needed in order to provide appropriate care.
Pender Health Promotion Model	Individuals will seek health promotion experiences in order to improve their well-being.

Essentials of Community Nursing

- A community is a group of people and institutions that share geographic, civic, and/or social parameters.

- Communities vary in their characteristics and health needs.

- A community's health is determined by the degree to which the community's collective health needs are identified and met.

- Health indicators (mortality rates, disease prevalence, levels of physical activity, obesity, tobacco use, substance abuse) are often used to describe the health status of a community and serve as targets for the improvement of a community's health.

- Community health nurses are nurses who practice in the community. They usually have a facility from which they work (community health clinic, county health department), but their practice is not limited to institutional settings.

- The community or a population (an aggregate who shares one or more personal characteristics) within the community is the "client" in community health nursing.

- Community partnership occurs when community members, agencies, and businesses actively participate in the processes of health promotion and disease prevention. The development of community partnerships is critical to the accomplishment of health promotion and disease prevention strategies.

- In population-focused nursing, assessments are made and interventions are provided for defined "at risk" populations (individuals with hypertension, individuals with nutrition and/or weight problems).

	FOCUS OF CARE	NURSING ACTIVITIES	LEVEL OF PREPARATION
Community-Oriented Nursing	• Health of the community as a "whole" • Client: Community	Health care: Surveillance and evaluation of the community's collective health, and the implementation of strategies to promote health and prevent disease	Generalist (bachelor of science in nursing) or specialist (master's degree in community or public health nursing)
Community-Based Nursing	• Health of individuals, families, and groups within a community • Client: Individual, family, or group of individuals	Illness care: Provision of direct primary care in the settings where individuals and families live, work, and "attend" (schools, camps, parishes)	Generalist (bachelor of science in nursing) or specialist (master's degree in maternal-infant nursing, pediatric nursing, adult nursing, mental health nursing)

	THEORY BASE	GOALS AND FUNCTIONS
Community Health Nursing Practice	Synthesis of nursing and public health theory	• Promote, preserve, and maintain the health of populations by the delivery of health services to individuals, families, and groups in order to impact "community health."

	THEORY BASE	GOALS AND FUNCTIONS

Health Nursing tice	Synthesis of nursing and public health theory	• Promote, preserve, and maintain the health of populations through disease and disability prevention and health protection of the community as a whole.
		• Core functions are:
		  o Systematic assessment of the health of populations
		  o Development of policies to support the health of populations
		  o Ensuring that essential health services are available to all persons

PRINCIPLES OF COMMUNITY HEALTH NURSING

 Overview

- Principles guiding community health nursing practice include:

  o Ethical Considerations

  o Advocacy

  o Epidemiology

  o Epidemiological Calculations

  o Epidemiological Triangle

  o The Epidemiological Process

  o Community-Based Health Education

Ethical Considerations

- The Public Health Code of Ethics identifies the ethical practice of public health. Ethical considerations include preventing harm, doing no harm, promoting good, respecting both individual and community rights, respecting autonomy and diversity, and providing confidentiality, competency, trustworthiness, and advocacy.

- Community health nurses are concerned with protecting, promoting, preserving, and maintaining health, as well as preventing disease. These concerns reflect the ethical principle of promoting good and preventing harm. Balancing individual rights versus rights of community groups is a challenge.

- Community health nurses address the challenges of autonomy and providing ethical care. Client rights include the right to information disclosure, privacy, informed consent, information confidentiality, and participation in treatment decisions.

APPLICATION OF ETHICAL PRINCIPLES TO COMMUNITY HEALTH NURSING		
ETHICAL PRINCIPLES	DEFINITION	COMMUNITY HEALTH NURSING SITUATIONS
Respect for Autonomy	Individuals select those actions that fulfill their goals.	Client's right to self-determination (making a decision not to pursue chemotherapy)
Nonmaleficence	No harm is done when applying standards of care.	Developing plans of care that include a system for monitoring and evaluating outcomes
Beneficence	Maximize possible benefits and minimize possible harms.	Assessment of risk and benefits
Distributive Justice	Fair distribution of the benefits and burden in society is based on the needs and contributions of its members.	Determining who will be eligible for health care services based on income and fiscal resources

Advocacy

- One role of the community health nurse is that of the advocate. The nurse plays the role of informer, supporter, and mediator for the client. The following are basic to client advocacy.

    ○ Clients are autonomous beings who have the right to make decisions affecting their own health and welfare.

    ○ Clients have the right to expect a nurse-client relationship that is based on trust, collaboration, and shared respect, related to health, and considerate of their thoughts and feelings.

    ○ Clients are responsible for their own health.

    ○ It is the nurse's responsibility to ensure access to services that meet the client's health care needs.

    ○ In order to be an advocate for the client, the nurse must be assertive, recognize that the values of the client and family must be a priority even when they conflict with health care providers, and intervene politically if necessary.

Epidemiology

- Epidemiology is the investigative study of disease trends in populations for the purposes of disease prevention and health maintenance.

- Epidemiology relies on statistical evidence to determine the rate of spread of disease and the proportion of people affected. It also is used to evaluate the effectiveness of disease prevention and health promotion activities and to determine the extent to which their goals have been met.

- Epidemiology is useful for community-based nursing in providing a broad understanding of the spread and transmission of disease. This information often forms the basis of community health presentations.

Epidemiological Triangle

SUSCEPTIBLE INDIVIDUALS (HOSTS)

- Altered immunity
- Altered resistance
- Risk characteristics
  - Genetics
  - Gender
  - Age
  - Physiological state
  - Prior disease state
  - Social class
  - Cultural group
  - Occupation

INTERMEDIARY (LIVING) VECTORS

- Mosquitos
- Fleas
- Rodents
- Birds
- Ticks

INFECTIOUS AGENTS

- Viruses
- Fungi
- Bacteria
- Protozoa
- Metazoa
- Rickettsia

PHYSICAL AGENTS

- Trauma
- Genetics
- Noise
- Temperature
- Repetitive motions

CHEMICAL AGENTS

- Drugs
- Fumes
- Toxins

NONSUSCEPTIBLE INDIVIDUALS (HOSTS)

- Active immunity
  - Natural
  - Artificial
- Passive immunity
  - Natural
  - Artificial

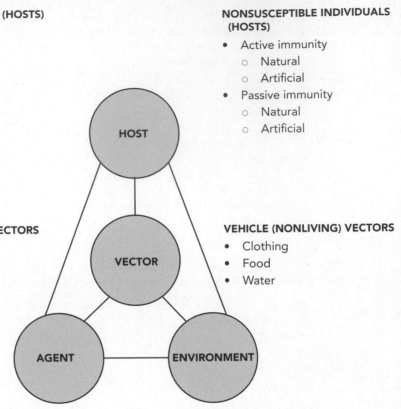

VEHICLE (NONLIVING) VECTORS

- Clothing
- Food
- Water

ENVIRONMENTAL RESERVOIRS AND MODES OF TRANSMISSION

- Human reservoirs
- Physical factors
- Temperature
- Rainfall
- Socioeconomic factors
- Availability of resources
- Access to health care
- High-risk working conditions
- Crowded living conditions

- Using the scientific problem-solving method, the nurse is able to pinpoint health needs in the community and develop appropriate approaches. Community health nurses are in the unique position of being able to identify cases, recognize patterns of disease, eliminate barriers to disease control, and provide education and counseling targeted at a disease condition or specific risk factors.

- Epidemiology involves the study of the relationships among an agent, a host, and an environment (referred to as the epidemiological triangle). Their interaction determines the development and cessation of communicable diseases, and they form a web of causality, which increases or decreases the risk for disease.

  o The agent is the animate or inanimate object that causes the disease.

  o The host is the living being that will be affected by the agent.

  o The environment is the setting or surrounding that sustains the host.

Epidemiological Calculations

- Incidence (new cases)

  o Number of cases in the population at a specific time ÷ population total x 1,000 = _____ per 1,000

- Prevalence (existing disease in a population at a particular time)

  o Number of cases in the population at a specific time ÷ population total x 1,000 = _____ per 1,000

- Crude Mortality Rate

  o Number of deaths ÷ population total x 1,000 = _____ per 1,000

- Infant Mortality Rate

  o Number of infant deaths before 1 year of age in a year ÷ numbers of live births in the same year x 1,000 = _____ per 1,000

- Attack Rate

  o Number of people at risk who develop a certain disease ÷ total # of people at risk

- An epidemic is when the rate of disease exceeds the usual level of the condition.

The Epidemiological Process

PHASE	DESCRIPTION
Determine the nature, extent, and possible significance of the problem.	During this phase of the process, the nurse collects information from as many sources as possible. This information is then used to determine the scope of the problem.
Using the gathered data, formulate a possible theory.	At this time, the nurse projects and explores the possible explanations.
Gather information from a variety of sources in order to narrow down the possibilities.	The nurse assesses all possible sites for amassing information related to the disease process. The nurse evaluates the plausibility of the proposed hypothesis.
Make the plan.	In this phase of the process, the nurse focuses on breaking the cycle of disease. All factors influencing the spread of the disease must be considered and identified. Priorities are established to break the chain of transmission and to control the spread of the disease.
Put the plan into action.	Using all available means, the nurse puts the plan for controlling the disease into action.
Evaluate the plan.	The nurse gathers pertinent information to determine the success of the plan. Using this plan, the nurse evaluates the success in prevention of the spread of the disease.
Report and follow up.	The nurse synthesizes evaluation data into a format that is understandable. Then nurse evaluates successes and failures and bases follow-up on the evaluation information.

Community-Based Health Education

- Community health nurses regularly provide health education in order to promote, maintain, and restore the health of populations. This is accomplished through a variety of means, such as community education programs.

- In designing community education programs, nurses must take into account the barriers that make learning difficult. Some of these obstacles include age, cultural barriers, poor reading and comprehension skills, language barriers, barriers to access, and lack of motivation. Effective community health education requires planning.

- Learning Theories Used in Community Health Nursing

    o Behavioral theory – Focus is on changing behavior through the use of reinforcement methods.

    o Cognitive theory – Focus is on changing thought patterns through the use of methods that offer a variety of sensory input and repetition.

    o Critical theory – Focus is on increasing depth of knowledge through the use of methods such as discussion and inquiry.

- ○ Developmental theory – Focus is on the human developmental stage and methods that are age-specific and age-appropriate with importance given to "readiness to learn."

- ○ Humanistic theory – Focus is on feelings and relationships, and methods are based on the principle that learners will do what is in their best interests.

- ○ Social learning theory – Focus is on changing the learners' expectations and beliefs through the use of methods that link information to beliefs and values.

- Learning Styles

  - ○ Learning styles should be addressed in order to adequately provide education to the public.

    - ■ Visual learners learn through "seeing" and methods such as note taking, video viewing, and presentations. These learners "think in pictures."

    - ■ Auditory learners learn through "listening" and methods such as verbal lectures, discussion, and reading aloud. These learners "interpret meaning while listening."

    - ■ Tactile-kinesthetic learners learn through "doing" and methods such as trial and error, hands-on approaches, and return demonstration. These learners gain "meaning through exploration."

- Development of a Community Health Education Plan

  - ○ First, identify population-specific learning needs. Set priorities and select the priority learning need to be addressed.

  - ○ Select aspects of learning theories (behavioral, cognitive, critical, developmental, humanistic, social learning) to use in the educational program based on the identified learning need.

  - ○ Consider educational issues such as population-specific concerns, barriers to learning, and learning styles (visual, auditory, tactile-kinesthetic).

  - ○ Design the educational program.

    - ■ Set short- and long-term learning objectives that are measurable and achievable.

    - ■ Select an appropriate educational method based on learning objectives and assessment of participants' learning styles.

    - ■ Select content appropriate to learning objectives and allotted time frame.

    - ■ Select an evaluation method that will provide feedback regarding achievement of short-term learning objectives.

  - ○ Implement the education program. Ensure an environment that is conducive to learning (minimal distractions, favorable to interaction, learner comfort, readability).

  - ○ Evaluate the achievement of learning objectives and the effectiveness of instruction.

HEALTH PROMOTION AND DISEASE PREVENTION

Overview

- National health goals guide the nurse in developing health promotion strategies to improve individual and community health.

- Community health nurses participate in three levels of prevention – primary, secondary and tertiary.

Health Promotion

- National health goals are derived from scientific data and trends collected during the prior decade. These goals are based on those issues that are considered major risks to the health and wellness of the United States' population.

  o *Healthy People* was initiated in 1979, and every 10 years, publishes the national health objectives that serve as a guide for promoting health and preventing disease.

  o *Healthy People* is coordinated by the United States Department of Health and Human Services, along with other federal agencies, and transitioned to *Healthy People 2020* in January of 2010.

- National health goals guide the nurse in developing health promotion strategies to improve individual and community health.

- The community health nurse actively helps people to change their lifestyles in order to move toward a state of optimal health (physical and psychosocial health).

- Preventive services include health education and counseling, immunizations, and other actions that aim to prevent a potential disease or disability.

- The community health nurse provides preventive services in multiple community settings.

- The community health nurse is often responsible for planning and implementing screening programs for at-risk populations.

- Successful screening programs provide accurate, reliable results, can be inexpensively and quickly administered to large groups, and produce few if any side effects.

 View Media Supplement: Levels of Prevention (Video)

Disease Prevention

LEVELS OF PREVENTION	EXAMPLES OF COMMUNITY HEALTH NURSE PREVENTION ACTIVITIES
Primary Prevention Focus – Prevention of the initial occurrence of disease or injury	• Nutrition counseling • Family planning and sex education • Smoking cessation education • Communicable disease education • Education about health and hygiene issues to specific groups (day care workers, restaurant workers) • Safety education (seatbelt use, helmet use) • Prenatal classes • Providing immunizations • Community assessments • Disease surveillance (communicable diseases) • Advocating for the resolution of health issues (access to health care, healthy environments)

Secondary Prevention
Focus – Early detection of disease and treatments with the goal of limiting severity and adverse effects
	• Screenings
	  ○ Cancer (breast, cervical, testicular, prostate, colorectal)
	  ○ Diabetes mellitus
	  ○ Hypertension
	  ○ Hypercholesterolemia
	  ○ Sensory impairments
	  ○ Tuberculosis
	  ○ Lead exposure
	  ○ Genetic disorders/metabolic deficiencies in newborns
	• Treatment of sexually transmitted diseases
	• Treatment of tuberculosis
	• Control of outbreaks of communicable diseases

Tertiary Prevention Focus – Maximization of recovery after an injury or illness (rehabilitation)	• Nutrition counseling • Exercise rehabilitation • Case management (chronic illness, mental illness) • Shelters • Support groups • Exercise for hypertensive clients (individual)

CHAPTER 1: OVERVIEW OF COMMUNITY HEALTH NURSING

(A) Application Exercises

1. Describe the events of the 1800s that impacted the community health care evolution.

2. Match the following historical figures with their contributions to community health nursing.

_____	Lillian Wald	A. Developed the Frontier Nursing Service
_____	Clara Barton	B. Developed the Red Cross
_____	Florence Nightingale	C. Established the Henry Street Settlement House
_____	Mary Breckinridge	D. Developed nursing training after returning from the war

3. The principle of autonomy includes which of the following? (Select all that apply.)

_____ Protection of privacy

_____ Respect for person

_____ Egalitarian approach

_____ Informed consent

_____ Fulfillment of client goals

Scenario: A toddler is seen at the clinic with the following clinical symptoms – Fever of 103, runny nose, dry cough, blotchy, reddish-brown rash, and white spots with blue centers inside the mouth (Koplik's spots). The child's provider reports the rash started on the face and progressed downward to the feet following a family trip to Switzerland. The child is diagnosed with measles. The next week, three more children present with similar symptoms, and are diagnosed with measles as well. Upon further investigation, it is found that all three children are in the same daycare class as the first child that was diagnosed. Of all four children, none had received the MMR immunization.

4. Who/what is the agent?

5. Who/what is the host?

6. Who/what is the environment (reservoir/mode of transmission)?

CHAPTER 1: OVERVIEW OF COMMUNITY HEALTH NURSING

 Application Exercises Answer Key

1. Describe the events of the 1800s that impacted community health care evolution.

> The Sisters of Mercy provided care for disadvantaged people. Florence Nightingale trained as a nurse in Germany and then established a training school for nurses in England. The city of New Orleans developed a department to address the need for quarantine and to look at the tuberculosis epidemic. Clara Barton established the Red Cross. Lillian Wald established the Henry Street Settlement.

 NCLEX® Connection: Management of Care: Advocacy

2. Match the following historical figures with their contributions to community health nursing.

__C__	Lillian Wald	A. Developed the Frontier Nursing Service
__B__	Clara Barton	B. Developed the Red Cross
__D__	Florence Nightingale	C. Established the Henry Street Settlement House
__A__	Mary Breckinridge	D. Developed nursing training after returning from the war

NCLEX® Connection: Management of Care: Advocacy

3. The principle of autonomy includes which of the following? (Select all that apply.)

__X__	**Protection of privacy**
__X__	**Respect for person**
_____	Egalitarian approach
__X__	**Informed consent**
__X__	**Fulfillment of client goals**

> Autonomy is the capacity to be one's own person and to live one's life according to self-determined reasons and motives that are not the product of external forces. Recognizing a client's autonomy displays respect for person, protects client rights (including the right to privacy), ensures informed consent, and allows for the fulfillment of client goals.

NCLEX® Connection: Management of Care: Advocacy

Scenario: A toddler is seen at the clinic with the following clinical symptoms – Fever of 103, runny nose, dry cough, blotchy, reddish-brown rash, and white spots with blue centers inside the mouth (Koplik's spots). The child's provider reports the rash started on the face and progressed downward to the feet following a family trip to Switzerland. The child is diagnosed with measles. The next week, three more children present with similar symptoms, and are diagnosed with measles as well. Upon further investigation, it is found that all three children are in the same daycare class as the first child that was diagnosed. Of all four children, none had received the MMR immunization.

4. Who/what is the agent?

The rubeola virus is the agent. Agents are biological, chemical, or physical. They can be bacteria, viruses, fungi, pesticides, food additives, psychological factors, or radiation. Some agents are transmitted to hosts by vectors; characteristics of agents include infectivity, pathogenicity and virulence.

 NCLEX® Connection: Physiological Adaptation: Alterations in Body Systems

5. Who/what is the host?

The infected children are the hosts. The host is a living organism capable of being infected or affected by the agent under natural conditions. The initial host was the first child seen in the clinic, who had likely already transmitted the virus to other children in the daycare. The hosts are more susceptible due to the fact that none had yet received the MMR immunization, and it is likely that any passive immunity provided from the children's mothers at birth is no longer effective. The age of the children also puts them at greater risk, as they are exploring their environment and often placing items in their mouths that might have been previously contaminated with the agent by another child.

 NCLEX® Connection: Physiological Adaptation: Alterations in Body Systems

6. Who/what is the environment (reservoir/mode of transmission)?

The environment is all that is external to the host, including how the agent was transmitted. In this scenario, the environment includes the human reservoir, the travel of the child to Switzerland, and the daycare setting that allowed for transmission of the virus to other children.

 NCLEX® Connection: Physiological Adaptation: Alterations in Body Systems

CHAPTER 2: FACTORS INFLUENCING COMMUNITY HEALTH

NCLEX® CONNECTIONS

When reviewing the content in this chapter, keep in mind the relevant sections of the NCLEX® outline, in particular:

CLIENT NEEDS: MANAGEMENT OF CARE

Relevant topics/tasks include:
- Continuity of Care
  - Maintain continuity of care between/among health care agencies.

CLIENT NEEDS: HEALTH PROMOTION AND MAINTENANCE

Relevant topics/tasks include:
- Aging Process
  - Assess client reactions to expected age-related changes.
- Developmental Stages and Transitions
  - Recognize cultural and religious influences that may impact family functioning.
- Health Promotion/Disease Prevention
  - Identify risk factors for disease/illness.

CLIENT NEEDS: PSYCHOSOCIAL INTEGRITY

Relevant topics/tasks include:
- Cultural Diversity
  - Respect the cultural background/practices of the client.

Chapter 2	Factors Influencing Community Health

Overview

- Factors that influence community health include family and cultural values, social and environmental influences, and economic concerns.

- Culture is defined as beliefs, values, and assumptions about life that are widely held among a group of people and are transmitted across generations.

- Environmental health refers to the influence of environmental conditions on the development of disease or injury.

- Community health nurses are responsible for increasing access to health care for vulnerable populations, such as children, older adults, clients who are physically/mentally disabled, unemployed, or homeless.

Family and Cultural Care

- Congruency between culture and health care is essential to the well-being of the client. The link between health beliefs and practices is greatly influenced by an individual's culture.

- It is important to assess cultural beliefs and practices when determining a plan of care.

  o Community health nurses need to consider that not all cultures are similar, and there are variations within each culture.

  o The uniqueness of each client needs to be considered.

  o Likewise, it is important for community health nurses to become familiar with cultures represented within the local community.

- Acculturation is the process of learning a new culture. Adapting to a new culture requires changes in daily living practices. These changes relate to language, education, work, recreation, social experiences, and the health care system.

- Cultural awareness includes self-awareness of one's own cultural background, biases, and differences. Health care professionals need to assess their own beliefs and consider how personal beliefs may affect the care given to clients.

- Meeting cultural needs of the client should be considered as important as meeting physical and psychological needs. Personal cultural values should not be imposed on the client, and nurses should be certain to avoid ethnocentrism and stereotyping in the provision of care.

- Cultural competence is knowing, appreciating, and considering the culture of someone else in resolving problems.

Cultural Assessment

- A cultural assessment provides information to the health care provider about the effect of culture on communication, space and physical contact, time, social organization, biologic variation, and environmental control factors.

  - General cultural-assessment parameters

    - Ethnic background

    - Religious preferences

    - Family structure

    - Language

    - Communication needs

    - Education

    - Cultural values

    - Food patterns

    - Health practices

  - The three steps of data collection

    - Collection of self-identifying data

    - Posing questions that address the client's perceptions of his health needs

    - Identification of cultural factors that may impact the choice of nursing interventions

Using an Interpreter

- An interpreter should be used when it is difficult for a nurse or client to understand the other's language.

- It is recommended to select an interpreter who has knowledge of health-related terminology. The use of family members as interpreters is generally not advisable, because clients may need privacy in discussing sensitive matters.

- Health teaching materials should be available in the client's primary language.

- The federal government mandates agencies have a plan to improve access to federal health care programs to individuals with limited English proficiency.

Cultural Competence: Areas for Self-Assessment

- Am I aware of my culture and views about other cultures?

- Am I able to do a culturally sensitive assessment?

- Do I have the knowledge necessary to develop nursing interventions?

- What is my experience in working with diverse populations?

- What is my goal in learning about diverse populations?

Conveying Cultural Sensitivity

- The nurse should:

  o Address clients by their last names, unless the client gives the nurse permission to use other names.

  o Introduce himself by name and explain his position.

  o Be authentic and honest about what he does or does not know about a client's culture.

  o Use language that is culturally sensitive.

  o Find out what clients know about their health problems and treatments, and assess cultural congruence.

  o Not make assumptions about clients.

  o Encourage clients to ask about anything that they may not understand.

  o Respect clients' values, beliefs, and practices.

  o Show respect for clients' support systems.

Environmental Risks

- Toxins such as lead, pesticides, mercury, air pollution, solvents, asbestos, and radon

- Air pollution such as carbon monoxide, particulate matter, ozone, lead, aerosols, nitrogen dioxide, sulfur dioxide, and tobacco smoke

- Water pollution such as wastes, erosion after mining or timbering, run-off from chemicals added to the soil

Roles for Nurses in Environmental Health

- Community involvement and public participation such as organizing community participation in decisions, informing, and facilitating discussions

- Individual and Population Risk Assessment

- Risk Communication

- Epidemiological Investigations

- Policy Development

Assessment of Environmental Health

- "I Prepare" Model

  - I = Investigate potential exposures

  - P = Present work (exposures, use of personal protective equipment, location of material safety data sheets [MSDS], taking home exposures, trends)

  - R = Residence (age of home, heating, recent remodeling, chemical storage, water)

  - E = Environmental concerns (air, water, soil, industries in neighborhood, waste site or landfill nearby)

  - P = Past work (exposures, farm work, military, volunteer, seasonal, length of work)

  - A = Activities (hobbies, activities, gardening, fishing, hunting, soldering, melting, burning, eating, pesticides, alternative healing/medicines)

  - R = Referrals and resource (Environmental Protection Agency, Agency for Toxic Substances & Disease Registry, Association of Occupational and Environmental Clinics, MSDS, OSHA, local health department, environmental agency, poison control)

  - E = Educate (risk reduction, prevention, follow-up)

- Key Questions for Environmental Health History

  - Housing: What is the physical condition of residence, age, location, school, day care, or work site? Are lighting, ventilation, and heating/cooling systems adequate?

  - What are the occupations of household members (current and past, longest-held jobs)?

  - Is tobacco smoke present?

  - Are there any recent home remodeling activities, such as the installation of new carpet or furniture or refinishing of furniture?

  - What hobbies are done in the home?

  - Is there any other recent exposure to chemicals or radiation?

  - Are pets present in the home, and are they healthy?

  - Has there been any lead exposure in old paint, crafts, leaded pottery, or dishes?

  - What is the source and quality of the drinking water?

  - How is sewage and waste disposed of in the home?

  - Are there pesticides used around the home or garden? Is there any evidence of mold or fungi?

  - Where do children play? Is there any hazardous play equipment or toys?

  - Does the surrounding neighborhood present any hazards with closeness to highways or small businesses, such as dry cleaning, photo processing, industry, or auto repair?

National Health Care Goals

- Reductions in:
    - Proportion of people exposed to air pollutants
    - Toxic air emissions
    - Waterborne disease outbreaks
    - Per capita domestic water use
    - Number of beach closings
    - Potential human exposure to persistent chemical by decreasing fish-contaminated levels
    - Pesticide exposures
    - Amount of toxic pollutants used for energy recovery
    - Indoor allergen levels
- Increases in:
    - Use of alternative modes of transportation to reduce motor-vehicle emissions
    - Nation's air quality
    - Proportion of people served by community water systems receiving a drinking water supply that meets Safe Drinking Water Act regulations
    - Proportion of rivers and lakes that are safe for fishing
    - Recycling of waste
    - Eliminate elevated blood levels of lead in children.

Environmental Health Nursing Interventions

LEVEL OF PREVENTION	INDIVIDUAL INTERVENTIONS	COMMUNITY INTERVENTIONS
Primary Prevention	• Educate individuals to reduce environmental hazards.	• Educate individuals to reduce environmental hazards. • Advocate for safe air and water. • Support programs for waste reduction and recycling. • Advocate for waste reduction and effective waste management.

LEVEL OF PREVENTION	INDIVIDUAL INTERVENTIONS	COMMUNITY INTERVENTIONS
Secondary Prevention	• Survey for health conditions that may be related to environmental and occupational exposures. • Obtain environmental health histories of individuals. • Monitor workers for levels of chemical exposures at job sites. • Screen children 6 months to 5 years old for blood lead levels.	• Survey for health conditions that may be related to environmental and occupational exposures. • Assess homes, schools, work sites, and the community for environmental hazards.
Tertiary Prevention	• Refer homeowners to lead abatement resources. • Educate asthmatic clients about environmental triggers.	• Become active in consumer and health-related organizations and legislation related to environmental health issues. • Support cleanup of toxic waste sites and removal of other hazards.

Access to Health Care

- Access to health care is impacted by more than availability of services in a community. The multifaceted impacts of individual, family, and community circumstances all influence access to health care.

- Community assessment includes evaluating the adequacy of health services within the community and the accessibility of those services by those needing access.

- Barriers to health care include:

    ○ Inadequate health care insurance

    ○ Inability to pay for health care services

    ○ Language barriers

    ○ Cultural barriers

    ○ Lack of health care providers in a community

    ○ Geographic isolation

    ○ Social isolation

    ○ Lack of communication tools (e.g., telephones)

    ○ Lack of personal or public transportation to health care facilities

    ○ Inconvenient hours

- o Attitudes of health care personnel toward clients of low socioeconomic status or those with different cultural/ethnic backgrounds

- o Eligibility requirements for state/federal assistance programs

- Community health nurses advocate for the accessibility of health care services

Health Care Organizations and Financing

- International Health Organizations

  - o World Health Organization (WHO)

    - Provides daily information regarding the occurrence of internationally important diseases.

    - Establishes world standards for antibiotics and vaccines.

    - The WHO primarily focuses on the health care workforce and education, environment, sanitation, infectious diseases, maternal and child health, and primary care.

- Federal Health Agencies

  - o U.S. Department of Health & Human Services

    - Under the direction of the secretary of health

    - Funded through federal taxes

    - Consists of 12 agencies

      - □ Administration for Children and Families

      - □ Administration on Aging

      - □ Centers for Medicare and Medicaid Services – also administers the Health Insurance Portability and Accountability Act (HIPAA), disability insurance, Aid to Families with Dependent Children (AFDC), and Supplemental Security Income (SSI).

MEDICARE	MEDICAID
• Medicare provides hospital and medical insurance to individuals who are 65 years and older, permanently disabled, and/or have end-stage renal failure. • Part A (hospital care, home care, limited skilled nursing care) • Part B (medical care, diagnostic services, physiotherapy) • Part C (also known as the Medicare Advantage plan – is a combination of Part A and Part B and is provided through a private insurance company) • Part D (prescription drug coverage)	• Medicaid provides financial assistance to states and counties to pay for health care services for older adults with low socioeconomic status, clients with disabilities, and families with dependent children. • Medicaid provides inpatient and outpatient hospital care, laboratory and radiology services, physician services, skilled nursing care at home or in a nursing home for persons older than 21 years, and early periodic screening, diagnosis, and treatment for those younger than 21 years.

- □ Agency for Healthcare Research and Quality

- □ Centers for Disease Control and Prevention - Works to prevent and control disease, injury, and disability both nationally and internationally.

- □ Agency for Toxic Substances and Disease Registry

- □ Food and Drug Administration

- □ Health Resources and Service Administration - Includes the Division of Nursing and the Divisions of Medicine, Dentistry, and Allied Health Professions.

- □ Indian Health Service

- □ National Institutes of Health - Supports biomedical research and includes the National Institute of Nursing Research.

- □ Substance Abuse and Mental Health Services Administration

- □ Office of the Secretary

- ○ Veterans Health Administration (within the U.S. Department of Veterans Affairs) - finances health services for active and retired military persons and dependents.

- • State Health Departments

  - ○ State departments of public health nursing, which manage the Women, Infants, and Children (WIC) program, are part of state health departments.

  - ○ State Children's Health Insurance Program (SCHIP) - offers expanded health care coverage to uninsured children.

  - ○ Board of Examiners of Nurses

    - ■ State Practice Act

    - ■ Licensing and examination of registered and licensed practical nurses (in some states known as licensed vocational nurses)

- ■ Approval/oversight of schools of nursing
- ■ Revocation, suspension, or denial of nursing licenses
- o Establishment of public health codes
- o Assistance/support for local health departments
- o Funded through state taxes and federal funding
- o Administration of Medicaid programs
- o Nursing roles: advocate, teacher, coordinator, and consultant

- Local Health Department

  - o The primary focus of a local health department is the health of its citizens.
  - o Local health departments offer various services and programs.
  - o The local community health nurse typically provides direct services such as referring caregivers of family members who are terminally ill to respite care and/or hospice services.
  - o Local health departments are funded through local taxes with support from federal and state funds.
  - o Nursing roles: advocate, teacher, coordinator, and consultant

- Private Funding

  - o Health insurance
  - o Employer benefits
  - o Managed care
    - ■ Health maintenance organizations (HMOs) - Comprehensive care is provided to members by a set of designated providers.
    - ■ Preferred provider organizations (PPOs) - Predetermined rates are set for services delivered to members; financial incentives are in place to promote use of PPO providers.
    - ■ Medical savings accounts - Untaxed money is put in an account for use for medical expenses.

CHAPTER 2: FACTORS INFLUENCING COMMUNITY HEALTH

 Application Exercises

1. A male client from Japan does not make eye contact with a nurse when she speaks. This nonverbal behavior is indicative of which of the following?

    A. The client has low self-esteem.

    B. The client is exhibiting signs of fatigue.

    C. The client has a negative attitude toward the nurse.

    D. Further assessment is needed of the client's culture and his feelings before a determination can be made.

2. An older adult woman from Croatia has been diagnosed with grade 4 breast cancer. She agrees that her family should be told that she has cancer, but she feels that information regarding the severity of her diagnosis should be withheld. Which of the following reflects a culturally sensitive nursing intervention?

    A. Contact an ethics committee to resolve the situation.

    B. Arrange for hospice care.

    C. Telling the client to get her "affairs" together.

    D. Establish a meeting with the client, family, and health team to discuss the client's diagnosis per the client's guidelines.

3. Which of the following are responsibilities of local health departments? (Select all that apply.)

    _____ Drug approval and control

    _____ Assessment of the health status of populations

    _____ Coordination of directives from state and federal levels

    _____ Determination of how well community health needs are being met

    _____ Licensing of registered nurses

4. A community health nurse is speaking with a 64-year-old client who recently moved to the state and has no health insurance. The client is a veteran and lives on a limited income. What can the nurse tell him about his options for health insurance?

5. A community health nurse is speaking with a young adult mother of two children who has just lost her job. She previously had health insurance through her employer. What can the nurse tell her about options for health insurance?

CHAPTER 2: FACTORS INFLUENCING COMMUNITY HEALTH

 Application Exercises Answer Key

1. A male client from Japan does not make eye contact with a nurse when she speaks. This nonverbal behavior is indicative of which of the following?

    A. The client has low self-esteem.

    B. The client is exhibiting signs of fatigue.

    C. The client has a negative attitude toward the nurse.

    D. Further assessment is needed of the client's culture and his feelings before a determination can be made.

It is important to avoid assumptions about the client's feelings and culture. Further assessment will provide greater insight into how to interpret his avoidance of eye contact.

NCLEX® Connection: Psychosocial Integrity: Cultural Diversity

2. An older adult woman from Croatia has been diagnosed with grade 4 breast cancer. She agrees that her family should be told that she has cancer, but she feels that information regarding the severity of her diagnosis should be withheld. Which of the following reflects a culturally sensitive nursing intervention?

    A. Contact an ethics committee to resolve the situation.

    B. Arrange for hospice care.

    C. Telling the client to get her "affairs" together.

    D. Establish a meeting with the client, family, and health team to discuss the client's diagnosis per the client's guidelines.

It is important to respect the client's values, beliefs, and practices. This is not an issue for an ethics committee, and it is not appropriate for the nurse to arrange for hospice care. Telling the client to get her affairs in order is a nontherapeutic response.

NCLEX® Connection: Psychosocial Integrity: Cultural Diversity

3. Which of the following are responsibilities of local health departments? (Select all that apply.)

    _____   Drug approval and control

    __**X**__   **Assessment of the health status of populations**

    __**X**__   **Coordination of directives from state and federal levels**

    __**X**__   **Determination of how well community health needs are being met**

    _____   Licensing of registered nurses

Local health departments are responsible for assessment of the health status of populations within their community and determining if the health needs of the community are being met. Local health departments are funded by federal and state taxes and therefore must coordinate directives from those levels. Approval and control of drugs is the responsibility of the Food and Drug Administration, which is a federal health agency. Licensing of registered nurses takes place at the state level.

 NCLEX® Connection: Management of Care: Continuity of Care

4. A community health nurse is speaking with a 64-year-old client who recently moved to the state and has no health insurance. The client is a veteran and lives on a limited income. What can the nurse tell him about his options for health insurance?

Because the client is a veteran, he could receive health care services through the Veterans Health Administration. He may also be eligible for Medicaid services, which are provided by each state. When the client turns 65, he will be eligible for Medicare, which is a national health insurance plan for older adults.

 NCLEX® Connection: Management of Care: Continuity of Care

5. A community health nurse is speaking with a young adult mother of two children who has just lost her job. She previously had health insurance through her employer. What can the nurse tell her about options for health insurance?

The Child Health Insurance Program (CHIP) provides expanded Medicaid coverage to children. They may also qualify for Medicaid benefits depending on the eligibility requirements of their state. The nurse should also make the client aware of the Health Insurance Portability and Accountability Act (HIPAA) of 1996, which is intended to provide health insurance coverage to people who lose their jobs.

 NCLEX® Connection: Management of Care: Continuity of Care

CHAPTER 3: COMMUNITY HEALTH PROGRAM PLANNING

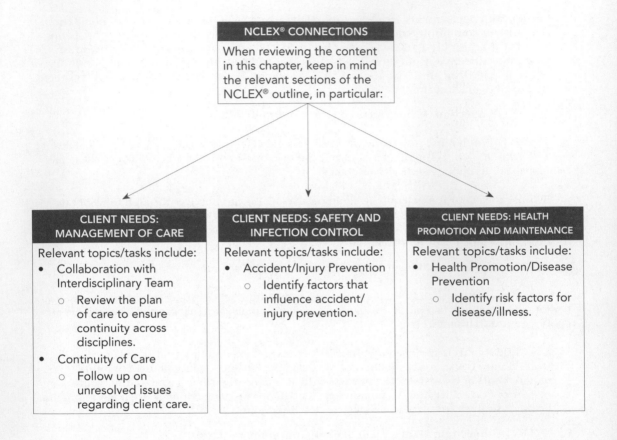

NCLEX® CONNECTIONS

When reviewing the content in this chapter, keep in mind the relevant sections of the NCLEX® outline, in particular:

CLIENT NEEDS: MANAGEMENT OF CARE

Relevant topics/tasks include:
- Collaboration with Interdisciplinary Team
  - Review the plan of care to ensure continuity across disciplines.
- Continuity of Care
  - Follow up on unresolved issues regarding client care.

CLIENT NEEDS: SAFETY AND INFECTION CONTROL

Relevant topics/tasks include:
- Accident/Injury Prevention
  - Identify factors that influence accident/injury prevention.

CLIENT NEEDS: HEALTH PROMOTION AND MAINTENANCE

Relevant topics/tasks include:
- Health Promotion/Disease Prevention
  - Identify risk factors for disease/illness.

Chapter 3   Community Health Program Planning

Overview

- The role of the community health nurse in community health program planning and evaluation is a collaborative leadership role. The desired outcome is to plan, organize, implement, and evaluate intervention programs that address the specific health needs of the community.

- Community health program planning should reflect the priorities set as a result of analysis of community assessment data. Priorities are established based on the extent of the problem (percent of population affected by the problem), the relevance of the problem to the public (degree of risk, economic loss), and the estimated impact of intervention (improvement of health outcome, adverse effects).

Community Assessment: Individual, Family, Community

- Community assessment is a comprehensive approach that identifies the community as a client.

- Community assessment and diagnosis are the foundation for population-specific program planning.

- Using the nursing process, nurses can determine health needs within the community and assist in developing and implementing strategies to meet those needs. In doing this, it is necessary to expand the assessment, diagnosis, planning, intervention, and evaluation efforts from the individual to the community or aggregate level.

- The community health nurse is a key player in assessing the needs of the community. This role includes:

  o   Interacting with community partners serving the community at large.

  o   Witnessing the interaction between community programs and the response of the client to the services.

  o   Identifying future services based upon the visible needs of population groups.

- Components of a Community Assessment

  o   People

    ▪   Demographic - Distribution, mobility, density, census data

    ▪   Biological factors - Health and disease status, genetics, race, age, gender, causes of death

- Social factors - Occupation, activities, marital status, education, income, crime rates, recreation, industry
- Cultural factors - Positions, roles, history, values, customs, norms, religion
  - Place or environment
    - Physical factors - Geography, terrain, type of community, location of health services, housing, animal control
    - Environmental factors - Geography, climate, flora, fauna, topography, toxic substances, vectors, pollutants
  - Social systems
    - Health systems
    - Economic systems/factors
    - Education systems
    - Religious systems
    - Welfare systems
    - Political systems
    - Recreation systems/factors
    - Legal systems
    - Communication systems/factors
    - Transportation systems
    - Resources and services

Data Collection

- Data collection is a critical community health nursing function. To best identify the health needs of the local community it is essential to combine several methods of data collection. Relying on only one or two key pieces can result in an incomplete assessment.

DATA COLLECTION METHOD	DESCRIPTION	STRENGTHS	LIMITATIONS
Informant Interviews	Direct discussion with community members for the purpose of obtaining ideas and opinions from key informants	• Minimal cost • Participants serving as future supporters	• Built-in bias • Meeting time and place
Community Forum	Open public meeting	• Opportunity for community input • Minimal cost	• Difficulty finding a convenient time and place • Potential to drift from the issue • Challenging to get adequate participation • Possibility that a less vocal person may be reluctant to speak
Secondary Data	Use of existing data (death statistics, birth statistics, census data, mortality, morbidity data) to assess problem	• Database of prior concerns/needs of population • Ability to trend health issues over time	• Possibility that data may not represent current situation • Can be time consuming
Windshield Survey	Descriptive approach that assesses several community components by driving through a community	• Provides a descriptive overview of a community	• Need for a driver so the nurse can visualize and document the community elements • May be time consuming • Results based only on visualization and does not include input from community members

DATA COLLECTION METHOD	DESCRIPTION	STRENGTHS	LIMITATIONS
Focus Groups	Directed talk with a representative sample	• Minimal cost • Possibility of participants being potential supporters • Provides insight into community support	• Possible discussion of irrelevant issues • Challenging to get participants • Difficult to ensure that sample is truly representative of the overall community
Surveys	Specific questions asked in a written format	• Data collected on client population and problems • Random sampling	• Low response rate • Expensive • Time consuming • Possibility of the collection of superficial data
Participant Observation	Observation of formal or informal community activities	• Indication of community priorities, environmental profile, and identification of power structures	• Bias

- Windshield Survey Components
  - People
    - Who is on the street?
    - How are they dressed?
    - What are they doing?
    - What is the origin, ethnicity, or race of the people?
    - How are the different groups (subgroups) residentially located?
    - How should the nurse categorize the socioeconomic status of the residents? Why?
    - Is there any evidence of drug abuse, violence, disease, mental illness? If yes, why does the nurse think so?
    - Are there any animals or pets in the community?
  - Place
    - Boundaries
      - Where is the community located?
      - What are its boundaries?
      - Are there natural boundaries?
      - Are there human-made boundaries?

- Location of health services
  - □ Where are the major health facilities located?
  - □ What health care facilities are necessary for the community but are not within the community?

- Natural environment
  - □ Are there geographic features that may harm the community?
  - □ Are there plants or animals that could harm or threaten the health of the community?

- Human-made environment
  - □ What industries are within the communities?
  - □ Could these pose a threat to the health of community workers or the community itself?
  - □ Is there easy access to health care facilities?
  - □ Are the roads adequate and marked well?

- Housing
  - □ Is the housing of acceptable quality?
  - □ How old are the homes?
  - □ Are there single or multifamily dwellings?
  - □ Is the housing in good repair or disrepair?
  - □ Is there vacant housing? Why?

- Social systems
  - □ Are there social services, clinics, hospitals, dentists, and health care providers available within the community?
  - □ Are there ample schools within the community? Are they in good repair or disrepair?
  - □ Are there parks or areas for recreation?
  - □ What places of worship are within the community?
  - □ What services are provided by local religious groups, schools, community centers, and activity or recreation centers?
  - □ Is there public transportation? Is it effective?
  - □ What grocery stores or other stores are within the community?
  - □ Is public protection evident (police, fire, EMS services)?

Analysis of Community Assessment Data

- The community health nurse plays an active role in assessment, data interpretation, and problem identification. Steps in analysis of community assessment data include:

    o Gathering collected data into a composite database.

    o Assessing completeness of data.

    o Identifying and generating missing data.

    o Synthesizing data and identifying themes.

    o Identifying community needs and problems.

    o Identifying community strengths and resources.

- Problem analysis is completed for each identified problem. Frequently, work groups are formed to examine individual problems and develop solutions.

- In the problem statement, the nurse should identify expected outcomes based on specific and measurable criteria.

Community Health Diagnoses

- Problems identified by community assessments are often stated as community health diagnoses.

- Community nursing diagnoses incorporate information from the community assessment, general nursing knowledge, and epidemiological concepts (especially the concept of risk in a population).

- Community nursing diagnoses often are written in the following format:

    o Risk of (specific problem or risk in the community) among (the specific population that is affected by the problem or risk) related to (strengths and weaknesses in the community that influence the problem or risk).

Community Health Program Planning

- In setting priorities among identified community problems, factors to be considered include:

    o Community awareness of the problem

    o Community readiness to acknowledge and address the problem

    o Available expertise/fiscal resources

    o Severity of the problem

    o Amount of time needed for problem resolution

PLANNING PHASES	DESCRIPTION	ACTIVITIES	COMMUNITY HEALTH NURSING ROLE
Preplanning	Brainstorm ideas.	Obtain community awareness, support, and involvement.	• Collaborate in developing a problem statement, goal statement, and timeline. • Assess resources and develop interventions with community partners. • Coordinate collaborations that have similar interests in addressing identified problems.
Assessment	Collect data about the population.	Evaluate the trends and risk factors of the population for the identified health need.	• Complete a needs assessment and identify community strengths. • Develop priorities and establish outcomes.
Policy Development	Plan interventions to meet identified outcomes, focusing on education, enforcement, and engineering elements.	Establish methods for allocating the resources and ascertaining rights, status, and resources.	• Initiate interventions to meet outcomes by linking resources to needs, developing community partnerships, and planning interventions that impact health protection and promotion and disease prevention. • Determine funding opportunities for needed interventions.
Implementation	Carry out the plan.	Identify the sequence of interventions and when they should occur.	• Monitor the intervention process and the response of the community in terms of its values, needs, and perceptions.
Evaluation	Examine the success of the interventions.	Document the progress of the interventions, compare the outcomes against a standard, and modify the interventions based on results.	• Modify the interventions to meet the needs of the population. • Share findings with population groups.

Development of a Plan for a Community Health Program

- Establish goals and objectives. Generally, the goal is to decrease the incidence and prevalence of the identified problem. Objectives are behaviorally stated, measurable, and include a target date for achievement.

- Select strategies/interventions to meet the objectives.

- Plan a logical sequence for interventions by establishing a timetable.

- Identify who will assume responsibility for each intervention.

- Assess the personnel needed and any special training they may require for screening or providing education.

- Assess supplies, equipment, educational materials, office space, locations for screenings, and educational services.

- Develop a budget.

- Plan for program evaluation.

- Implement the program.

- Evaluate the program.

Strategies and Barriers in Implementing Community Health Programs

HELPFUL STRATEGIES	BARRIERS
Thorough assessment	Inadequate assessment
Accurate interpretation of data	Inadequate or misconstrued data
Collaboration with community partners	No involvement with community partners
Effective communication patterns	Impaired communication
Sufficient resources	Inadequate resources
Logical planning	Lack of planning
Skilled leadership	Poor leadership

Community Health Program Evaluation

- It is important to remember that evaluation is an ongoing process.

- Program evaluation should document not only success in meeting outcomes but also the efficiency and effectiveness of the program plan and specific interventions.

- Because a multitude of variables impact health outcomes in a community, it is often difficult to measure all of the variables and interventions used to address the issue.

- Evaluation is needed throughout the program to respond to the changing needs of the population.

- Results of evaluation efforts should always be reported to key team members, as well as the community members. Be certain information provided to the community is provided in terminology that can be easily understood.

CHAPTER 3: COMMUNITY HEALTH PROGRAM PLANNING

 Application Exercises

1. Identify strategies for successful implementation of health programs.

2. Identify barriers for successful implementation of health programs.

3. A community health nurse is evaluating a community health program designed to promote car safety for infants. The program was implemented 2 years ago. Explain how the nurse should identify appropriate program evaluation steps.

4. Directed conversation with select members of a community about a health problem is the data assessment method known as

    A. key informant interviews.

    B. participant observation.

    C. focus groups.

    D. windshield survey.

5. Which of the following are examples of sources for secondary data? (Select all that apply.)

    _____ Birth statistics

    _____ Death statistics

    _____ Previous health survey results

    _____ Minutes from past community meetings

    _____ Windshield survey

    _____ Community forum

    _____ Health records

6. A community health nurse collects data for a community assessment. The following information is noted about the community:

    Low crime rate
    Weekly curbside garbage pick-up
    Small amount of litter along the road
    Public transportation that operates 24 hr a day, 7 days a week
    Many opportunities for residents to be active in the community, including several community organizations
    Recreational trails that are in need of maintenance and repair

What methods were most likely used to collect these data?

CHAPTER 3: COMMUNITY HEALTH PROGRAM PLANNING

 Application Exercises Answer Key

1. Identify strategies for successful implementation of health programs.

> **Successful implementation of health programs requires accurate assessment of need, active involvement of community participants in identifying the health problem, adequate resources, logical planning, community partnerships, and leadership.**

 NCLEX® Connection: Management of Care: Continuity of Care

2. Identify barriers for successful implementation of health programs.

> **Barriers for successful implementation of health programs include poor assessment, disagreement of what the health problem is, lack of leadership, lack of resources, insufficient community involvement, and poor planning.**

 NCLEX® Connection: Management of Care: Continuity of Care

3. A community health nurse is evaluating a community health program designed to promote car safety for infants. The program was implemented 2 years ago. Explain how the nurse should identify appropriate program evaluation steps.

> **Determine if the program goals and objectives were met. Pose questions ("How many parents attended the educational program about infant car seat safety?"). Identify the number of correctly installed car seats. Compare/contrast rates of prior car seat use with current rates and investigate if there has been a decline in infant injury or death related to changes in the use of car seats.**

> **Gather feedback by asking parents questions ("What was helpful about the car safety program?", "What areas should be improved?", "Overall, were you satisfied with the program?", "Might you recommend the program to other parents?").**

 NCLEX® Connection: Safety and Infection Control: Accident /Injury Prevention

4. Directed conversation with select members of a community about a health problem is the data assessment method known as

> **A. key informant interviews.**
> B. participant observation.
> C. focus groups.
> D. windshield survey.

> **Informant interviews are direct discussions with community members for the purpose of obtaining ideas and opinions. Participant observation is the observation of formal or informal community activities. Focus groups are directed talk with a representative sample. Windshield survey is a descriptive approach that assesses several community components by driving through a community.**

 NCLEX® Connection: Management of Care: Collaboration with Interdisciplinary Team

5. Which of the following are examples of sources for secondary data? (Select all that apply.)

   __X__   **Birth statistics**

   __X__   **Death statistics**

   __X__   **Previous health survey results**

   __X__   **Minutes from past community meetings**

   _____   Windshield survey

   _____   Community forum

   __X__   **Health records**

Birth statistics, death statistics, previous health survey results, minutes from past community meetings, and health records are all sources for secondary data.

Windshield survey and community forum are data collection methods.

 NCLEX® Connection: Health Promotion and Maintenance: Health Promotion/Disease Prevention

6. A community health nurse collects data for a community assessment. The following information is noted about the community:

Low crime rate

Weekly curbside garbage pick-up

Small amount of litter along the road

Public transportation that operates 24 hr a day, 7 days a week

Many opportunities for residents to be active in the community, including several community organizations

Recreational trails that are in need of maintenance and repair

What methods were most likely used to collect these data?

Likely methods include (but are not limited to):

Low crime rate: Obtaining statistics at city hall (secondary data)

Weekly curbside garbage pick-up: Interviewing the city mayor (informant interview)

Small amount of litter along the road: Driving through the community (windshield survey)

Public transportation that operates 24 hr a day, 7 days a week: Interviewing the city mayor (informant interview)

Many opportunities for residents to be active in the community, including several community organizations: Interviewing a parent-teacher association (focus group)

Recreational trails that are in need of maintenance and repair: Driving through the community (windshield survey)

 NCLEX® Connection: Health Promotion and Maintenance: Health Promotion/Disease Prevention

CHAPTER 4: PRACTICE SETTINGS AND AGGREGATES

NCLEX® CONNECTIONS

When reviewing the content in this chapter, keep in mind the relevant sections of the NCLEX® outline, in particular:

CLIENT NEEDS: SAFETY AND INFECTION CONTROL

Relevant topics/tasks include:
- Accident/Injury Prevention
  - Identify deficits that may impede client safety.
- Handling Hazardous and Infectious Materials
  - Follow procedures for handling biohazardous materials.
- Standard Precautions/ Transmission-Based Precautions/Surgical Asepsis
  - Follow correct policy and procedures when reporting a client with a communicable disease.

CLIENT NEEDS: HEALTH PROMOTION AND MAINTENANCE

Relevant topics/tasks include:
- Health and Wellness
  - Assess client perception of health status.
- Health Promotion/Disease Prevention
  - Assess and teach the client about health risks based on known population or community characteristics.
- High-Risk Behaviors
  - Assist the client to identify behaviors/ risks that may impact health.

CLIENT NEEDS: PSYCHOSOCIAL INTEGRITY

Relevant topics/tasks include:
- End of Life Care
  - Provide end of life care and education to clients.
- Religious and Spiritual Influences on Health
  - Assess psychosocial, spiritual, and occupational factors affecting care and plan interventions, as appropriate.

Chapter 4	Practice Settings and Aggregates

Overview

- Community health nurses practice in a diverse range of settings.
- Community health nurses practice as:
    - Home health nurses
    - Hospice nurses
    - Occupational health nurses
    - Parish nurses
    - School nurses
    - Case managers
- The aggregates that receive services from community health nurses include:
    - Individuals from infancy to death
    - Families
    - Groups within the community
- It is important to be aware of health disparities of each group and to minimize those disparities if possible.

Practice Settings

- Home Health Nurse
    - Community health nurses provide care in the home. This is a means for providing health care services to clients where they reside. This includes traditional homes, assisted living facilities, and nursing homes.
    - Multidisciplinary care is essential to care for the client holistically.
        - Nurses, physical therapists, occupational therapists, home health aides, social workers, and dietitians may be part of the interdisciplinary care provided in the home.
        - These services are prescribed by a primary care provider and usually overseen by a nurse.

- o The home health nurse functions as educator, provider of skilled nursing interventions, and coordinator of care.
  - Many clients leave the hospital in just a few days and are still very ill.
  - These clients and their family members need skilled services and education about the disease process, prescribed medications, and future implications of their illnesses.
- o Home health nurses provide a variety of skilled services, including, but not limited to:
  - Skilled assessment
  - Wound care
  - Laboratory draws
  - Medication education and administration
  - Parenteral nutrition
  - IV fluids and medication
  - Central line care
  - Urinary catheter insertion and maintenance
  - Coordination/supervision of various other participants in health services
- o The home health nurse must evaluate the living environment for safety, paying close attention to non secure rugs, electrical outlets, and extension cords, the use of oxygen, safety devices in the bathroom, and other potential environmental hazards.
  - Older adult are at a particular risk for falls.
  - Nurses should ask the following questions:
    - □ Does the client have food in the house to eat?
    - □ Is there help with household activities?
    - □ Does the client live alone?
    - □ Who is the client's support system?
    - □ Is the client able to set up and dispense his own medication?
    - □ Does the client have access to health care?
- o Home health nurses often provide follow-up care after an acute hospital stay; therefore, they must educate the client and the family regarding complications or adverse reactions.
  - These instructions may include when to contact the agency, the emergency room, or the provider. Information and resources for families and clients can provide support in dealing with illness.
- o By providing clients with education about their diseases, nurses encourage clients to be independent and to be involved in their own care. It also allows the family to be involved in the care and decision-making regarding their family member.

- Hospice Nurse

  o Hospice care, also known as palliative care, can be provided in a variety of settings including the home, hospice centers, hospitals, and long-term care settings.

  o Hospice care is a comprehensive care delivery system for the terminally ill that is usually implemented when the client is not expected to live longer than 6 months. Further medical care aimed towards cure is stopped and the focus becomes relief of pain and suffering, and enhancing quality of life.

  o Care is provided for the client, as well as the client's entire family.

  o Hospice care uses an interdisciplinary approach.

  o Controlling symptoms is a priority.

  o Hospice care services are directed by the provider and managed by the nurse.

  o Volunteers are used for nonmedical care.

  o Postmortem bereavement services are offered for the family.

  o Helping the family transition from an expectation of recovery to acceptance of death is an important aspect of providing hospice care. The hospice nurse may continue to work with the family for up to 1 year following the death of the client.

- Occupational Health Nurse

  o The occupational health nurse works towards the health and safety of workers by:

    ▪ Assessing risks for work-related illness and injury.

    ▪ Planning and delivery of health and safety services in the workplace.

    ▪ Facilitating health promotion activities that lead to a more productive workforce.

  o This autonomous specialty entails making independent nursing judgments when providing care to the workforce aggregate.

  o In assessing risk for work-related illness and injury, the nurse should keep in mind the following factors affecting susceptibility to illness and injury:

    ▪ Host factors:

      □ Worker characteristics, such as job inexperience, age, and pregnancy.

    ▪ Agent factors:

      □ Biological agents (viruses, bacteria, fungi, bloodborne, airborne pathogens)

      □ Chemical agents (asbestos, smoke)

      □ Mechanical agents (musculoskeletal or other strains from repetitive motions, poor workstation-worker fit, lifting heavy loads)

      □ Physical agents (temperature extremes, vibrations, noise, radiation, lighting)

      □ Psychological agents (threats to psychological or social well-being resulting in work-related stress, burnout, violence).

- Environmental factors:
    - Physical factors (heat, odor, ventilation, pollution);
    - Social factors (sanitation, housing conditions, overcrowding, illiteracy);
    - Psychological factors (addictions, stress).
- Occupational health nurses' roles and responsibilities include:
    - Primary prevention - Teaching good nutrition and knowledge of health hazards, identifying workplace hazards, and providing information on immunizations, use of protective equipment, and smoking cessation.
    - Secondary prevention - Early detection through health surveillance and screening, prompt treatment, counseling and referral, and prevention of further limitations.
    - Tertiary prevention - Restoration of health through rehabilitation strategies and limited duty programs.
- An occupational health history provides the framework for a nurse to begin to assess a worker for possible exposure to health hazards.
    - The goal is to identify agents and host factors that place the worker at risk and to identify ways to eliminate or minimize exposure and prevent potential health problems.
    - Information elicited should include:
        - Current and past jobs
        - Current and past exposure to specific agents and any relationship of current symptoms to work activities
        - Any precipitating factors, such as underlying illness, previous injuries, and healthy and unhealthy habits
- A worksite walk-through or survey is also part of a workplace assessment. Focus should be given to:
    - Observation of work processes and materials.
    - Job requirements.
    - Actual and potential hazards.
    - Employee work practices (hygiene, waste disposal, housekeeping).
    - Incidence/prevalence of work-related illness/injuries.
    - Control strategies to eliminate exposures.
- Control strategies are designed to reduce future exposures based upon results from investigations into work-related illness/injury. Control strategies often include:
    - Engineering
    - Altering work practices
    - Providing personal protective equipment and education to prevent future injuries
    - Workplace monitoring

- Health screening
- Employee-assistance programs
- Job-task analysis
- Design, risk management, and emergency preparedness

- ○ Protection from violence
  - Work can be frustrating and can contribute to stress, resulting in aggression and violence against others.
  - Being aware of jobs that are repetitive, boring, or physically and psychologically draining can help to identify workers who may feel tired, angry, and generally inadequate.
  - Nurses can refer such workers to employee-assistance programs that provide confidential counseling and referrals to other professional services if needed.
- ○ Protection from work-related injuries from falls, environmental hazards, and burns
  - Nurses can use research and trend analysis to improve working conditions by eliminating or minimizing hazards and potential problems.
  - Additional strategies include:
    - □ Providing safety and health education programs to workers.
    - □ Developing health policy focused on ensuring effective employee health and safety.
    - □ Designing strategies to prevent work-related accidents/injuries.
    - □ Keeping abreast of Occupational Health and Safety Administration (OSHA) standards and resource programs.
    - □ Working to influence legislation aimed at workers/workplace health protection.
- School Nurse
  - ○ School nursing encompasses many roles:
    - Case manager: ensures the provision and evaluation of comprehensive school-based health services and other related services for the children.
    - Community outreach: strives to meet the needs of all school-age children by cooperative planning and collaboration between the educational system and other community agencies.
    - Consultant: assists students, families, and personnel in information gathering and decision-making about a variety of health needs and resources.
    - Counselor: supports students on a wide variety of health needs.
    - Direct caregiver: provides nursing care to ill or injured children at school.
    - Health educator: helps prepare children, families, school personnel, and the community to make well-informed health decisions.
    - Researcher: contributes to the base of knowledge for school health and educational needs.

LEVELS OF PREVENTION IN SCHOOL NURSING	
ASSESSMENTS	EXAMPLES OF NURSING INTERVENTIONS
Primary prevention	

Assess the knowledge base regarding health issues.	• Teach health promotion practices:
	  o Hand hygiene and tooth-brushing
	  o Healthy food choices
	  o Injury prevention including bike and water safety
	  o Substance abuse prevention

Assess the immunization status of all children.	• Maintain current records of required immunizations.
Secondary prevention	

Assess children who become ill or injured at school.	• Provide care to children with:
	  o Headaches
	  o Stomach pain
	  o Injuries that occur at school

Assess all children, faculty, and staff during emergencies.	• Provide emergency care such as first aid and CPR. • The school clinic should have commonly needed supplies.

Perform screening for early detection of disease.	• Screenings include:
	  o Vision and hearing
	  o Height and weight
	  o Oral health
	  o Scoliosis
	  o Infestations (Lice)
	  o General physical examinations

Assess children to detect child abuse or neglect.	• The school nurse is required by state law to officially report all suspected cases of child abuse/neglect.
Assess children for evidence of mental illness, suicide, and violence.	• Identify children at risk.

LEVELS OF PREVENTION IN SCHOOL NURSING	
ASSESSMENTS	EXAMPLES OF NURSING INTERVENTIONS
Tertiary prevention	
Assess children with disabilities.	• Participate in developing the individual education plan (IEP) for children with disabilities. • Work with child/family to develop and achieve long-term outcomes.

Assess children with long-term health needs at school.	• Provide nursing care for children with disorders including: asthma, diabetes mellitus, and cystic fibrosis.
	• Responsible for administering medication per the provider's prescription.
	• The prescribed medication should be in the original bottle and be stored in a secure place.
	• Written consent by the parents is required.
	• Provide care to children who have specific health needs, including:
	   o Urinary catheterizations
	   o Dressing changes
	   o IV line monitoring

COMPONENTS OF COMPREHENSIVE SCHOOL HEALTH PROGRAMS	
COMPONENT	DESCRIPTION
Health education	Teaching children concepts of health
Physical education	Promoting physical activity in school
Health services	Providing health services in school at an appropriate nurse-to-student ratio (1:750)
Nutrition services	Teaching nutrition and diet concepts and providing breakfast and lunch for children who qualify by federal standards
Counseling, psychological, and social services	Promoting health of children with special needs, including those who receive special education services through the Individuals with Disabilities Act (IDEA)
Promotion of a healthy school environment	Reducing tobacco use and violence in schools
Health promotion for staff	Providing health care for school teachers and staff
Facilitation of family/community involvement	Promoting health services in the community

Aggregates of the Community

- Children (Birth to 12 years) and Adolescents
    - Health concerns/leading causes of death
        - Children
            - Perinatal conditions/congenital anomalies
            - Sudden Infant Death Syndrome (SIDS)
            - Motor vehicle/other unintentional injuries
        - Adolescents
            - Motor vehicle/other unintentional injuries
            - Homicide
            - Suicide
    - Screening/preventive services
        - Children
            - Height/weight
            - Vision
            - At birth - Hemoglobinopathy, phenylalanine level, T4, and TSH
            - Immunization status - Check the Centers for Disease Control and Prevention (CDC) Web site, www.cdc.gov, for current administration schedules.
            - Dental health
        - Adolescents
            - Height/weight
            - Dental health
            - Papanicolaou (Pap) smear test (females)
            - Chlamydia screen (females)
            - Rubella serology/vaccination history (females)
            - Substance abuse
            - Immunization status (www.cdc.gov)
            - Mental health screenings
    - Health care goals
        - Children and adolescents
            - Reductions in:
                - Obesity
                - Passive smoking

- ☐ Increases in:
  - ▸ Childhood immunizations
  - ▸ Child safety restraints
  - ▸ Exercise in schools
  - ▸ Lead-based paint testing
- ○ Community education
  - ■ Children
    - ☐ Breastfeeding
    - ☐ Sleeping positions
    - ☐ Nutrition
    - ☐ Physical activity
    - ☐ Substance use
    - ☐ Dental hygiene/health
    - ☐ Skin protection
    - ☐ Injury prevention including car, fire, and water safety; helmet use; poison control; and CPR training
  - ■ Adolescents
    - ☐ Substance use
    - ☐ Sexual behavior
    - ☐ Nutrition, especially calcium intake for females
    - ☐ Physical activity
    - ☐ Skin protection
    - ☐ Injury prevention including car, fire, and firearm safety
- ● Women
  - ○ Health concerns/leading causes of death
    - ■ Reproductive health
      - ☐ Childbearing
      - ☐ Menopause
      - ☐ Osteoporosis
    - ■ Heart disease
    - ■ Diabetes mellitus
    - ■ Malignant neoplasm (breast, cervical, ovarian, colorectal)

- o Screening/preventive services
  - Height/weight
  - Blood pressure
  - Cholesterol (ages 45-64)
  - Dental health
  - Pap smear test
  - Mammogram/clinical breast exam
  - Fecal occult blood test/sigmoidoscopy (≥ 50 years)
  - Rubella serology/vaccination history (childbearing years)
  - Immunization status – check the CDC Web site, www.cdc.gov, for current administration schedules
  - Diabetes mellitus
  - HIV
  - Skin cancer
- o Health Care Goals
  - Reductions in:
    - Diseases involving bone such as osteoporosis
    - Death from cancer such as breast, ovarian, and cervical
    - Sexual assaults
  - Increases in:
    - Number of planned pregnancies versus unplanned
    - Those who receive early and adequate prenatal care
    - The number of mothers who breastfeed
    - Identification of warning signs related to heart disease
- o Community Education
  - Nutrition
  - STD prevention
  - Substance use
  - Breast self-examination
  - Skin protection
  - HIV prevention
  - Injury prevention including car, fire safety, and violence

- Men
  - Health concerns/leading causes of death
    - Heart disease
    - Malignant neoplasm (prostate, testicular, skin, colorectal)
    - Accidents
    - Lung disease
    - Liver disease
  - Screening/preventive services
    - Height/weight
    - Blood pressure
    - Dental health
    - Digital rectal exam
    - Fecal occult blood test/sigmoidoscopy ($\geq$ 50 years)
    - Immunization status – check the CDC Web site, www.cdc.gov, for current administration schedules
    - Diabetes mellitus
    - HIV
    - Skin cancer
    - Cholesterol (ages 35-64 years)
  - Health care goals
    - Reductions in:
      - Death from cancer specific to men, such as prostate
      - Incidence of HIV and AIDS
      - Death by violent means
    - Increases in:
      - The number of men who are actively involved in pregnancy prevention/ family planning
      - Identification of warning signs related to heart disease
  - Community education
    - Nutrition
    - Self-testicular exam
    - Skin protection
    - Substance use
    - HIV prevention
    - Injury prevention including car, fire and firearm safety, and violence

Ⓖ • Older Adults

- ○ Health concerns/leading causes of death
  - ▪ Heart disease
  - ▪ Malignant neoplasm
  - ▪ Cerebrovascular disease
  - ▪ Chronic obstructive pulmonary disease
  - ▪ Pneumonia and influenza
- ○ Screening/preventive services
  - ▪ Blood pressure
  - ▪ Height/weight
  - ▪ Dental health
  - ▪ Fecal occult blood test/sigmoidoscopy
  - ▪ Mammogram/clinical breast exam (women)
  - ▪ Pap smear test (women)
  - ▪ Vision
  - ▪ Hearing
  - ▪ Substance abuse
  - ▪ Immunization status (pneumococcal, influenza) – check the CDC Web site, www.cdc.gov, for current administration schedules
  - ▪ Functional assessment (self-care abilities)
  - ▪ Medication history
  - ▪ Osteoporosis
  - ▪ Diabetes mellitus
  - ▪ Skin cancer
- ○ Health care goals
  - ▪ Reductions in:
    - ▫ Number of adults with musculoskeletal concerns
    - ▫ Number of older adults who have mental health concerns
    - ▫ Hospitalizations due to cardiac issues
    - ▫ Substance use in the older adult
    - ▫ Sensory concerns such as hearing loss and cataracts
  - ▪ Increases in:
    - ▫ Review of medications to reduce polypharmacy
    - ▫ The number of older adults who maintain an active lifestyle

- ○ Community education
  - Substance use
  - Nutrition
  - Exercise
  - Dental health
  - Sexual behavior
  - Injury prevention
    - □ Car and fire safety
    - □ Fall prevention
    - □ CPR training (household members)
    - □ Violence
- Families
  - ○ The family as client is basic to community-oriented nursing practice. Community health nurses have a significant role to play in promoting healthy families.
  - ○ Community health nurses must engage in community assessment, planning, development, and evaluation activities that are focused on family issues.
  - ○ Home visits provide community health nurses with the opportunity to observe the home environment and to identify barriers and supports to health-risk reduction.
  - ○ Family crisis occurs when a family is not able to cope with an event. The family's resources are inadequate for the demands of the situation.
  - ○ Transitions are times of risk for families.
    - Transitions include birth or adoption of a child, death of a family member, child moving out of the home, marriage of a child, major illness, divorce, and loss of the main family income.
    - These transitions require families to change behaviors, make new decisions, reallocate family roles, learn new skills, and learn to use new resources.
  - ○ Characteristics of healthy families
    - Members communicate well and listen to each other.
    - There is affirmation and support for all members.
    - Members teach respect for others.
    - There is a sense of trust.
    - Members play and share humor together.
    - Members interact with one another.
    - There is a shared sense of responsibility.
    - There are traditions and rituals.
    - Members seek help for their problems.

- o Family health risk appraisal
  - Biological health risk assessment:
    - □ Genograms are used to gather basic information about the family, relationships within the family, and health and illness patterns.
    - □ Repetitions of diseases with a genetic component (cancer, heart disease, diabetes mellitus) can be identified.
  - Environmental risk: Ecomaps are used to identify family interactions with other groups and organizations. Information about the family's support network and social risk is gathered.
  - Behavioral risk: Information is gathered about the family's health behavior, including health values, health habits, and health risk perceptions.
- o Health care goals
  - Reductions in:
    - □ Barriers to access
    - □ Allergic content within the home
    - □ Number of families who are unable to have a child or maintain a pregnancy
    - □ Passive smoke exposure
  - Increases in:
    - □ The amount of agency-provided education on health related issues
    - □ Home testing for radon and lead
    - □ Number of hungry families

CHAPTER 4: PRACTICE SETTINGS AND AGGREGATES

Ⓐ Application Exercises

1. A community health nurse identifies the need for a community health education program regarding breast self-examination for a population of older adult women at a community wellness center. Most of the women speak Spanish as their primary language. The nurse decides to show a short video about breast self-examination followed by a discussion of the technique for breast self-examination. The nurse will also have a mannequin available for participants to use to practice breast self-examination techniques. What are potential educational issues to be considered specific to this population?

2. The philosophy of hospice care includes which of the following?

    A. Instruct the client on life-sustaining measures.

    B. Teach the family that diseases can be cured.

    C. Provide support for clients and families.

    D. Focusing on the specific disease process during care.

Scenario: A nurse has just started a new job as a school nurse. The school board has asked her to evaluate the school health program and suggest areas for improvement. When assessing the school health program, the nurse discovers the following:

- There is one school nurse for every 1,000 students.
- There is no wellness program for faculty and staff.
- The school is free of environmental hazards.
- There is no medication administration policy in place.
- The school works with a neighboring hospital and provides students with health care through a collaborative volunteer program.
- Complete clinical services are available at the school-based clinic during school hours.
- Physical education classes are offered twice a week for all students.
- The school provides a nutritionally balanced breakfast and lunch program.
- The school employs a full-time counselor.
- Health education that is planned is provided for students at each grade level by the school nurse.
- The school is a smoke-free environment.
- Two children who use wheelchairs are tutored at home and do not attend classes at the school.

3. What strengths and weaknesses are present in the school health program?

4. Which weakness in the school health program is the highest in priority and requires immediate change? Why?

5. A nurse is completing an occupational health history on a worker. What questions should the nurse include?

6. What elements should be included in a worksite assessment?

7. A client presents to the community health clinic for a free mammogram and Pap smear. She is a 45-year-old Hispanic female and has not received health care of any kind since the birth of her youngest child, who is now 10 years old. She was just hired for full-time employment and is in need of a complete physical examination as required for the position. The medical history provided by the client is unremarkable. She has no documentation of immunizations from her childhood. She says that she had varicella as a child. She reports five spontaneous vaginal deliveries. Her husband of 25 years died 6 months ago. Identify the health screenings that are recommended for this client.

8. A wellness screening and educational program is being offered at a local senior center in the Midwest during the month of October. The focus of the screening is on health promotion during the winter months. Identify some topics that should be considered for inclusion in the educational program.

CHAPTER 4: PRACTICE SETTINGS AND AGGREGATES

 Application Exercises Answer Key

1. A community health nurse identifies the need for a community health education program regarding breast self-examination for a population of older adult women at a community wellness center. Most of the women speak Spanish as their primary language. The nurse decides to show a short video about breast self-examination followed by a discussion of the technique for breast self-examination. The nurse will also have a mannequin available for participants to use to practice breast self-examination techniques. What are potential educational issues to be considered specific to this population?

In designing community education programs, nurses must take into account the barriers that make learning difficult. Some of these obstacles include age, cultural barriers, poor reading and comprehension skills, language barriers, and lack of motivation. The age of this population may pose some issues, such as perceptions of minimal benefits of early detection and possibly some sensory-perceptual alterations. Use of an interpreter and a video in Spanish may need to be considered.

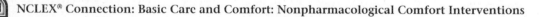 **NCLEX® Connection: Health Promotion and Maintenance: Health and Wellness**

2. The philosophy of hospice care includes which of the following?

A. Instruct the client on life-sustaining measures.

B. Teach the family that diseases can be cured.

C. Provide support for clients and families.

D. Focusing on the specific disease process during care.

The philosophy of hospice is to provide palliative care to terminally ill clients. The basis of palliative care is to support the client and family, and provide symptom control. Teaching life-sustaining measures and that diseases can be cured are not philosophies of hospice. The focus of hospice is to assist the client and family, through the efforts of an interdisciplinary team, in achieving the highest quality of life possible. Hospice does not focus on specific disease processes.

NCLEX® Connection: Basic Care and Comfort: Nonpharmacological Comfort Interventions

Scenario: A nurse has just started a new job as a school nurse. The school board has asked her to evaluate the school health program and suggest areas for improvement. When assessing the school health program, the nurse discovers the following:

- There is one school nurse for every 1,000 students.
- There is no wellness program for faculty and staff.
- The school is free of environmental hazards.
- There is no medication administration policy in place.
- The school works with a neighboring hospital and provides students with health care through a collaborative volunteer program.
- Complete clinical services are available at the school-based clinic during school hours.
- Physical education classes are offered twice a week for all students.
- The school provides a nutritionally balanced breakfast and lunch program.
- The school employs a full-time counselor.
- Health education that is planned is provided for students at each grade level by the school nurse.
- The school is a smoke-free environment.
- Two children who use wheelchairs are tutored at home and do not attend classes at the school.

3. What strengths and weaknesses are present in the school health program?

Strengths:

School is free of hazards and is smoke free.

There is collaboration with community agencies for health care.

Complete health services are available at the school, including a school counselor.

Physical education is provided at school.

Nutrition programs are in place for students.

Health education is given to students.

Weaknesses:

There is no medication administration policy.

There is no health promotion program for the staff.

The nurse-to-student ratio is too high.

Children with chronic illnesses are excluded from school.

 NCLEX® Connection: Health Promotion and Maintenance: Health and Wellness

4. Which weakness in the school health program is the highest in priority and requires immediate change? Why?

> The greatest weakness is the lack of a medication administration policy. In order to comply with federal and state laws that protect children, a policy should be developed immediately to safeguard the children who receive medication in the schools.

 NCLEX® Connection: Health Promotion and Maintenance: Health Promotion/Disease Prevention

---

5. A nurse is completing an occupational health history on a worker. What questions should the nurse include?

> **What type of work do you do?**
>
> **What potential exposures have you experienced?**
>
> **To what processes and operations, raw materials, and by-products are you exposed?**
>
> **What is your work environment like (e.g., general conditions, safety signs and precautions, physical environment, cleanliness, ventilation)?**
>
> **What work-related illnesses/injuries have you had?**
>
> **What is your average number of days missed per year and the reasons for those absences?**
>
> **What types of uniforms, clothing do you wear? How is it laundered?**

 NCLEX® Connection: Safety and Infection Control: Accident /Injury Prevention

6. What elements should be included in a worksite assessment?

> **The work, work processes, and related hazards, products, and exposures**
>
> **Work environment (cleanliness, clutter, ventilation, noise, temperature, lighting, safety, signs, waste disposal mechanisms)**
>
> **Worker population characteristics**
>
> **Staffing and personnel**
>
> **Corporate culture**
>
> **Written policies/procedures for occupational health care**
>
> **Most common illnesses/injuries**
>
> **Health promotion programs**
>
> **Regulatory compliance with OSHA standards**

 NCLEX® Connection: Safety and Infection Control: Accident /Injury Prevention

7. A client presents to the community health clinic for a free mammogram and Pap smear. She is a 45-year-old Hispanic female and has not received health care of any kind since the birth of her youngest child, who is now 10 years old. She was just hired for full-time employment and is in need of a complete physical examination as required for the position. The medical history provided by the client is unremarkable. She has no documentation of immunizations from her childhood. She says that she had varicella as a child. She reports five spontaneous vaginal deliveries. Her husband of 25 years died 6 months ago. Identify the health screenings that are recommended for this client.

Height

Weight

Blood pressure

Total blood cholesterol

Immunization status

Pap smear test

Baseline mammogram and clinical breast exam

Substance abuse

Dental health

(N) NCLEX® Connection: Health Promotion and Maintenance: Health Promotion/Disease Prevention

8. A wellness screening and educational program is being offered at a local senior center in the Midwest during the month of October. The focus of the screening is on health promotion during the winter months. Identify some topics that should be considered for inclusion in the educational program.

Prevention of falls, particularly related to weather conditions

Importance of influenza vaccines

Weather-related issues (staying warm, driving precautions)

Other general topics: nutrition, home safety, medication safety

(N) NCLEX® Connection: Health Promotion and Maintenance: Aging Process

CHAPTER 5: CARE OF SPECIAL POPULATIONS

- Violence
- Substance Abuse
- Mental Health
- Homelessness
- Rural and Migrant Health

NCLEX® CONNECTIONS

When reviewing the content in this chapter, keep in mind the relevant sections of the NCLEX® outline, in particular:

CLIENT NEEDS:
HEALTH PROMOTION AND MAINTENANCE

Relevant topics/tasks include:
- Developmental Stages and Transitions
  - Modify approaches to care in accordance with the client's developmental stage.
- Health and Wellness
  - Encourage client participation in appropriate behavior modification programs related to health and wellness.
- High-Risk Behaviors
  - Provide information for prevention of high-risk health behaviors.

CLIENT NEEDS:
PSYCHOSOCIAL INTEGRITY

Relevant topics/tasks include:
- Abuse/Neglect
  - Identify risk factors for domestic, child, elder abuse/neglect and sexual abuse.
- Chemical and Other Dependencies
  - Encourage the client to participate in support groups.
- Stress Management
  - Assess stressors, including environmental, that affect client care.

Chapter 5	Care of Special Populations

Overview

- Community health nurses care for many individuals who are members of special populations. These vulnerable populations include individuals who are subject to issues such as:

  o Violence

  o Substance abuse

  o Mental health

  o Homelessness

  o Rural and migrant health

- These individuals usually have difficulty accessing health care.

- Other factors that affect these individuals include:

  o Poverty

  o Poor self esteem

  o Young or advanced age

  o Chronic stress

  o Emotional instability

  o Environmental factors

- Health care goals to address for vulnerable populations include:

  o Encouraging people to use primary care providers for medical services.

  o Increasing the number of people with health insurance.

  o Making access to health care easier for the immigrant population.

VIOLENCE

- Types of Violence Within Communities

  o Homicide

    ▪ When committed by strangers, homicide is often related to a substance abuse network.

    ▪ Most homicides are committed by a friend, acquaintance, or family member during an argument.

- Within families, homicide is often preceded by abuse of a family member.
- Rates are increasing among adolescents.
- ○ Assault
  - Males are more likely to be assaulted.
  - Youths are at a significantly higher risk.
- ○ Rape
  - Rape is often unreported.
    - □ It includes date and marital rape.
    - □ The majority of violence against women is intimate partner violence.
    - □ There is an increased incidence reported in cities between the hours of 8 p.m. and 2 a.m., on weekends, and in the summer.
- ○ Suicide
  - More suicide attempts are reported for women.
  - Men are more likely to die from suicide.
  - Male adolescents, ages 15-19, are more likely to commit suicide than females in the same age range.
- ○ Abuse
  - Physical violence occurs when pain or harm results:
    - □ Toward an infant or child, as is the case with shaken baby syndrome (caused by violent shaking of young infants).
    - □ Toward a domestic partner, such as striking or strangling the partner.
    - □ Toward an older adult in the home (elder abuse), such as pushing an older adult parent and causing her to fall.
  - Sexual violence occurs when sexual contact takes place without consent, whether the victim is able or unable to give that consent.
  - Emotional violence, which includes behavior that minimizes an individual's feelings of self-worth or humiliates, threatens, or intimidates a family member.
  - Neglect includes the failure to provide:
    - □ Physical care, such as feeding
    - □ The emotional care and/or stimulation necessary for a child to develop normally, such as speaking and interacting with a child
    - □ An education for a child, such as enrolling a young child in school
    - □ Needed health or dental care
  - Economic Maltreatment
    - □ Failure to provide the needs of a victim when adequate funds are available
    - □ Unpaid bills when another person is managing the finances, resulting in disconnection of heat or electricity

- Individual Assessment for Violence
    - Factors influencing an individual's potential for violence
        - History of being abused or exposure to violence
        - Low self-esteem
        - Fear and distrust of others
        - Poor self-control
        - Inadequate social skills
        - Immature motivation for marriage or childbearing
        - Weak coping skills
- Recognizing Actual or Potential Child Abuse
    - Unexplained injury
    - Unusual fear of the nurse and others
    - Evidence of injuries not mentioned in history (old burns, scars, ecchymosis, human bite marks)
    - Fractures, including older healed fractures
    - Subdural hematomas
    - Trauma to genitalia
    - Malnourishment or dehydration
    - General poor hygiene or inappropriate dress for weather conditions
    - Considered to be a "bad child"
- Recognizing Potential or Actual Older Adult Abuse
    - Unexplained or repeated physical injuries
    - Physical neglect and unmet basic needs
    - Rejection of assistance by caregiver
    - Financial mismanagement
    - Withdrawal and passivity
    - Depression
- Community Assessment: Social and Community Factors Influencing Violence
    - Work stress
    - Unemployment
    - Media exposure to violence
    - Crowded living conditions
    - Poverty
    - Feelings of powerlessness
    - Social isolation
    - Lack of community resources (playgrounds, parks, theaters)

(S) • Strategies to reduce societal violence

PRIMARY PREVENTION	SECONDARY PREVENTION	TERTIARY PREVENTION
• Teach alternative methods of conflict resolution, anger management, and coping strategies in community settings. • Organize parenting classes to provide anticipatory guidance of expected age-appropriate behaviors, appropriate parental responses, and forms of discipline. • Educate clients about community services that are available to provide protection from violence. • Promote public understanding about the aging process and about safeguards to ensure a safe and secure environment for older adults in the community. • Assist in removing or reducing factors that contribute to stress by referring caretakers of older adult clients to respite services, assisting an unemployed parent in finding employment, or increasing social support networks for socially isolated families. • Encourage older adults and their families to safeguard their funds and property by getting more information about a financial representative trust, durable power of attorney, a representative payee, and joint tenancy. • Teach individuals that no one has a right to touch or hurt another person, and make sure they know how to report cases of abuse.	• Identify and screen those at risk for abuse and individuals who are potential abusers. • Assess and evaluate any unexplained bruises or injuries of any individual. • Screen all pregnant women for potential abuse. This may be the one time in some women's lives that they may access the health care system on a regular basis. • Refer sexual assault or rape victims to a local emergency department for assessment by a sexual assault abuse team. Caution the client not to bathe following the assault because it will destroy physical evidence. • Assess and counsel anyone contemplating suicide or homicide and refer the individual to the appropriate services. • Support and educate the offender, even though a report must be made. • Assess and help offenders address and deal with the stressors that may be causing or contributing to the abuse, such as mental illness or substance abuse. • Alert all involved about available resources within the community.	• Establish parameters for long-term follow-up and supervision. • Make resources in the community available to the client (telephone numbers of crisis lines and shelters). • If court systems are involved, work with parents while the child is out of the home (in foster care). • Refer to mental health professionals for long-term assistance. • Provide grief counseling to families of suicide or homicide victims. • Develop support groups for caregivers and victims of violence. • Advocate for legislation designed to assist older adult independence and caregivers and to increase funding for programs that supply services to low-income, at-risk individuals.

- When caring for clients who experience violence:

  o Build trust and confidence with a client.

  o Focus on the client rather than the situation.

  o Assess for immediate danger.

  o Provide emergency care as needed.

  o Develop a plan for safety.

  o Make needed referrals for community services and legal options.

  o If abuse has occurred, complete mandatory reporting, following agency guidelines.

SUBSTANCE ABUSE

- Substance abuse is the use of any substance (including legal and prescribed) that threatens an individual's health or social and economic functioning.

- Substance abuse affects all family members and often produces codependency in the nonaddicted individuals in relationships with the addicted individual.

- Substance abuse harms family life, public safety, and the economy.

- Addiction is a pattern of pathological, compulsive use of substances that can involve physiological dependence.

  o Cardinal signs of addiction are tolerance and withdrawal.

  o Denial is also a primary sign of addiction and may include:

    ▪ Defensiveness

    ▪ Lying about use

    ▪ Minimizing use

    ▪ Blaming or rationalizing use

    ▪ Intellectualizing

- Alcohol, tobacco, and other drug abuse and addiction can cause multiple health problems, including:

  o Low birth weight

  o Congenital abnormalities

  o Accidents

  o Homicides

  o Suicides

  o Chronic diseases

  o Violence

- Recovery from substance addiction occurs over years and usually involves relapses. A strong support system, including 12-step programs and self-help groups for family members, is important.

- Community health nurses are front-line health professionals who are able to assist those with addiction.

- Alcohol Use

  o Alcohol is the most commonly used substance in the United States. It is socially acceptable, as well as easily accessible.

  o Alcohol is a depressant. Alcohol dulls the senses to outside stimulation and sedates the inhibitory centers in the brain.

  o The direct effect of alcohol is determined by the blood alcohol level.

    ▪ The body processes alcohol dependent on several factors, including:

      □ The size and weight of the drinker

      □ Gender (affects metabolism)

      □ Carbonation (increases absorption)

      □ Time elapsed during alcohol consumption

      □ Food in the stomach

      □ The drinker's emotional state

    ▪ Alcohol is filtered by the liver at about 1 oz per hr.

    ▪ Excess alcohol that is not metabolized circulates in the blood and affects the central nervous system and the brain.

  o People who frequently and consistently drink alcohol develop a tolerance, an increased requirement for alcohol to achieve the desired effect.

    ▪ When people continue to drink consistently, they can develop blackouts, which are times when they continue to appear to function but later cannot remember anything about those times.

  o Withdrawal from alcohol begins commonly about 6 hr after cessation of drinking.

    ▪ Withdrawal can manifest itself with:

      □ Irritability

      □ Tremors

      □ Nausea

      □ Vomiting

      □ Headaches

      □ Diaphoresis

      □ Anxiety

      □ Sleep disturbances

- Increased blood pressure and pulse may result, with pulse being the clearest indicator of possible delirium tremens or alcohol withdrawal delirium.

- The prompt use of benzodiazepines at the onset of symptoms can prevent the serious complication of delirium tremens.

- It is important to determine the last drink the client has taken in order to accurately assess for signs of withdrawal and delirium tremens.

- Tobacco Use

  o Smoking is the most preventable cause of death in the United States, according to the Centers for Disease Control and Prevention.

  o Nicotine is a stimulant that temporarily creates a feeling of alertness and energy. Repeated use to avoid the subsequent "down" that will follow this period of stimulation leads to a vicious cycle of use and physical dependence (withdrawal effects if not consumed).

  o Tolerance to nicotine develops quickly.

  o Cigarette smoking results in deep inhalation of smoke, which poses the greatest health risk (cancer, cardiovascular disease, respiratory disease); however, cigars, pipes, and smokeless tobacco increase the risk of cancers of the lips, mouth, and throat. Secondhand smoke poses considerable health risks (respiratory disease, lung cancer) to nonsmokers.

- Other Drugs

  o Other stimulants include caffeine, amphetamines, and cocaine.

  o Other depressants include barbiturates, benzodiazepines, opioids, and heroin.

  o Hallucinogens (psychedelics) can produce euphoria, stimulation, and hallucinations. Some examples are lysergic acid diethylamide (LSD), phencyclidine (PCP), and MDMA (Ecstasy).

  o Inhalants are volatile substances that are inhaled ("huffed"). Death may result from acute cardiac dysrhythmias or asphyxiation.

- Individual Assessment

  o Establish rapport with the client. Pose questions in a matter-of-fact tone. Be nonjudgmental. Communicate that the purpose of questioning is because of the effects that different practices can have on an individual's health. Use the communication technique of normalizing when appropriate.

  o Seek information about specific substances used, methods of use, and the quantity (packs, ounces) and frequency of use.

  o Elicit information about consequences experienced (blackouts, overdoses, injuries to self/others, legal or social difficulties).

  o Determine if the individual perceives a substance abuse problem.

  o Discuss the individual's history of previous rehabilitation experiences.

  o Gather family history of substance abuse and social exposure to other substance users.

- ○ Some physical assessment findings include:

  - Vital signs – Blood pressure, pulse, and temperature can be elevated, while respirations can be rapid, shallow, and depressed.

  - Appearance – Individual can appear disheveled with an unsteady gait.

  - Eyes – Pupils can appear dilated or pinpoint, red, also poor eye contact.

  - Skin – Can be diaphoretic, cool, and/or clammy; needle track marks or spider angiomas may be visible.

  - Nose – Can be runny, congested, red and/or cauliflower-shaped.

  - Tremors – Fine or coarse tremors may be present.

- • Strategies to Reduce Substance Abuse

PRIMARY PREVENTION	SECONDARY PREVENTION	TERTIARY PREVENTION
• Increase public awareness, particularly among young people, regarding the hazards and addictive qualities of substance abuse (e.g., public education campaigns, school education programs). • Encourage development of life skills.	• Identify at-risk individuals and assist them to reduce sources of stress, including possible referral to social services to eliminate financial difficulties or other sources of stress. • Screen individuals for excessive substance use.	• Assist the client to develop a plan to avoid high-risk situations and to enhance coping and lifestyle changes. • Refer the client to community groups, such as Alcoholics Anonymous (AA) and Narcotics Anonymous (NA). • Monitor pharmacological management. • Provide emotional support to recovering abusers and their families, including positive reinforcement.

MENTAL HEALTH

- • Mental Illness Characteristics

  - ○ Occurs across the lifespan

  - ○ High risk of substance abuse

  - ○ High suicide risk

  - ○ Specific disorders include:

    - Affective disorders (bipolar disorder, major depression)

    - Anxiety disorders (obsessive-compulsive, panic, phobias, posttraumatic stress)

    - Schizophrenia

- - Dementia
  - Conduct disorders
  - Eating disorders
- Factors Contributing to Mental Health of Aggregates
  - o Individual coping abilities
  - o Stressful life events (exposure to violence)
  - o Social events (recent divorce, separation, unemployment, bereavement)
  - o Chronic health problems
  - o Stigma associated with seeking mental health services
- Strategies for Improving Mental Health

PRIMARY PREVENTION	SECONDARY PREVENTION	TERTIARY PREVENTION
• Educate populations regarding mental health issues. • Teach stress-reduction techniques. • Provide parenting classes. • Provide bereavement support. • Promote protective factors (coping abilities) and risk factor reduction.	• Screen to detect mental health disorders. • Work directly with individuals, families, and groups through the formation of a therapeutic relationship. • Conduct crisis intervention.	• Perform medication monitoring. • Provide mental health interventions. • Make referrals to various groups of professionals, including support groups. • Maintain the client's level of function to prevent relapse or frequent rehospitalization. • Identify behavioral, environmental, and biological triggers that may lead to relapse. • Assist the client in planning a regular lifestyle and minimizing sources of stress. • Educate the client and family regarding medication side effects, potential interactions

HOMELESSNESS

- Homeless Population Characteristics
  - o Adults who are unemployed, earn low wages, or are migrant workers
  - o Female heads of household
  - o Families with children (fastest growing segment)
  - o People who are mentally ill (large segment)

- People who abuse alcohol or other substances
- Abandoned children
- Adolescent runaways
- Older adults with no one to care for them

- Health Conditions of Homeless Populations

  - Upper respiratory disorders
  - Tuberculosis
  - Skin disorders (athlete's foot) and infestations (scabies, lice)
  - Alcoholism/drug abuse
  - HIV/AIDS
  - Assault and rape
  - Mental illness
  - Dental caries
  - Hypothermia and heat-related illnesses
  - Malnutrition

- Strategies for Preventing Homelessness and Assisting Individuals Who are Homeless

  - Prevent individuals and families from becoming homeless by assisting them in eliminating factors that may contribute to homelessness.
    - Refer those with underlying mental health disorders to therapy and counseling.
    - Enhance parenting skills that may prevent young people from feeling the need to run away.
  - Alleviate existing homelessness by making referrals for financial assistance, food supplements, and health services.
    - Assist homeless clients in locating temporary shelter.
    - Assist clients in finding ways to meet long-term shelter needs.
    - If homeless shelters are not provided in the community, work with government officials to develop shelter programs.
  - Prevent recurrence of poverty, homelessness, and health problems that result in conditions of poverty and homelessness.
    - Advocate and provide efforts toward political activity to provide needed services for people who are mentally ill and homeless.
    - Make referrals for employee assistance and educational programs to allow clients who are homeless to eliminate the factors contributing to their homelessness.

RURAL AND MIGRANT HEALTH

- Health Status of Rural Residents
  - Higher infant and maternal morbidity rates
  - Higher rates of chronic illnesses (heart, lung, hypertension, cancer, diabetes mellitus) and motor vehicle crash-related injuries
  - Higher health occupational risks (machinery accidents, skin cancer, respiratory problems due to chemical exposure)
  - Higher rates of suicide
  - High risk of trauma and injuries (falls, amputations, crush injuries, pesticide exposure)
  - Less likely to seek medical care
- Barriers to Health Care in Rural Areas
  - Distance from services
  - Lack of personal/public transportation
  - Unpredictable weather and/or travel conditions
  - Inability to pay for care/underinsured/uninsured
  - Shortage of rural hospitals/health care providers
- Health Problems of Migrant Workers
  - Dental disease
  - Tuberculosis
  - HIV
  - Depression and other mental health problems
  - Domestic violence
  - Lack of prenatal care
  - Higher infant mortality rates
- Issues in Migrant Health
  - Poor and unsanitary working and housing conditions
  - Less access to dental, mental health, and pharmacy services
  - Inability to afford care
  - Availability of services (distance, transportation, hours of service, health record tracking)
  - Language (majority speak Spanish) and cultural aspects of health care

- Strategies for Rural and Migrant Health Care

PRIMARY PREVENTION	SECONDARY PREVENTION	TERTIARY PREVENTION
• Educate regarding measures to reduce exposure to pesticides. • Teach regarding accident prevention measures. • Provide prenatal care. • Mobilize preventive services (dental, immunizations).	• Screen for pesticide exposure. • Screen for skin cancer. • Screen for chronic preventable diseases. • Screen for communicable diseases.	• Treat for symptoms of pesticide exposure. • Mobilize primary care and emergency services.

CHAPTER 5: CARE OF SPECIAL POPULATIONS

(A) Application Exercises

Scenario: A community mental health nurse is conducting a depression screening within a community. During the screening, the nurse assesses a 40-year-old client who has been divorced for 6 months. His two children, ages 13 and 15, are now living with their mother. The children refuse to talk to or see him. He has lost 20 lb since the divorce and says he lacks motivation to get out of the house to do anything besides go to work. He reports that he has difficulty falling asleep at night. He says he does not want to be labeled as "weird" for seeing a psychiatrist for mental health concerns.

1. What factors may be adversely affecting the mental health of this client?

2. What level of prevention is appropriate for interventions with this client at the screening? What are some examples of interventions at this level?

Scenario: A 19-year-old college freshman is seen at a community-based clinic for a follow-up exam for a broken leg, lacerations, and contusions. His chart reveals that these injuries were caused when the car he was driving hit a tree. His blood alcohol level was 0.189% 3 hr after the incident. He reports that he had spent the previous evening at a friend's apartment and had consumed a couple of beers. On his way home, he missed a turn and hit a tree. He sums it up as "no big deal."

3. What questions should the nurse ask to assess if the client is at risk for substance abuse?

4. What level of prevention is appropriate when working with this client at the clinic? What are examples of interventions at this level?

5. A community health nurse is working in a rural community. The nurse is to plan screenings and client education based on issues that affect the health of the rural community. Identify the health promotion and disease prevention screenings and education interventions that should be planned.

6. Name two health care goals that can be recommended for the immigrant population.

CHAPTER 5: CARE OF SPECIAL POPULATIONS

 Application Exercises Key

Scenario: A community mental health nurse is conducting a depression screening within a community. During the screening, the nurse assesses a 40-year-old client who has been divorced for 6 months. His two children, ages 13 and 15, are now living with their mother. The children refuse to talk to or see him. He has lost 20 lb since the divorce and says he lacks motivation to get out of the house to do anything besides go to work. He reports that he has difficulty falling asleep at night. He says he does not want to be labeled as "weird" for seeing a psychiatrist for mental health concerns.

1. What factors may be adversely affecting the mental health of this client?

> **The client's recent divorce and children not interacting with him could affect his mental health.**
>
> **The perceived stigma associated with seeking mental health services could also be a factor.**

NCLEX® Connection: Health Promotion and Maintenance: Health and Wellness

2. What level of prevention is appropriate for interventions with this client at the screening? What are some examples of interventions at this level?

> **Secondary prevention is appropriate. Specifically, the client needs to be screened for a mental health disorder. Some examples of secondary prevention interventions include identification of the illness in need of treatment (assessment), formation of a therapeutic relationship, and referral to necessary community resources.**

NCLEX® Connection: Health Promotion and Maintenance: Health Promotion/Disease Prevention

Scenario: A 19-year-old college freshman is seen at a community-based clinic for a follow-up exam for a broken leg, lacerations, and contusions. His chart reveals that these injuries were caused when the car he was driving hit a tree. His blood alcohol level was 0.189% 3 hr after the incident. He reports that he had spent the previous evening at a friend's apartment and had consumed a couple of beers. On his way home, he missed a turn and hit a tree. He sums it up as "no big deal."

3. What questions should the nurse ask to assess if the client is at risk for substance abuse?

> **Have you increased the amount of alcohol that you consume to obtain the effects that you used to have after a smaller amount of alcohol?**
>
> **Do you have a persistent desire to use alcohol?**
>
> **How often do you consume alcohol?**
>
> **Has your frequency of alcohol consumption increased or decreased over the past month?**
>
> **Have you missed classes or work because of use of alcohol?**

NCLEX® Connection: Psychosocial Integrity: Chemical and Other Dependencies

4. What level of prevention is appropriate when working with this client at the clinic? What are examples of interventions at this level?

> Secondary prevention is appropriate. Specifically, the client needs to be screened for a substance abuse problem. Some examples of secondary prevention interventions include:
>
>> Assess habits and history related to excessive alcohol consumption and use.
>>
>> In a nonjudgmental way, educate the client about the effects of alcohol, risks of drinking and driving, and the importance of preventing another motor vehicle crash.
>>
>> Explore the client's readiness and motivation to change his behavior.
>>
>> Explore alternative activities and college programs for recreation.
>>
>> If he chooses to make behavior changes, refer the client to a support group and/or counselor if necessary.
>>
>> If he chooses not to make immediate changes, encourage him to follow up with another appointment and to think about a decision that would promote health.

(N) NCLEX® Connection: Health Promotion and Maintenance: High Risk Behaviors

5. A community health nurse is working in a rural community. The nurse is to plan screenings and client education based on issues that affect the health of the rural community. Identify the health promotion and disease prevention screenings and education interventions that should be planned.

> Blood pressure
>
> Nutrition
>
> Diabetes mellitus
>
> Cholesterol
>
> Tobacco use
>
> Alcohol use or abuse
>
> Substance abuse
>
> Responsible use of prescription and over-the-counter medications
>
> Prenatal screenings and education
>
> Immunizations for all ages
>
> Cancer screenings (mammography, skin inspection, breast, testicular, Pap smears)
>
> Safety and exposure education

(N) NCLEX® Connection: Health Promotion and Maintenance: Health Screening

6. Name two health care goals that can be recommended for the immigrant population.

Encourage people to utilize providers for medical services, increase the number of people with health insurance, and make access to health care easier for immigrants.

Ⓝ **NCLEX® Connection: Health Promotion and Maintenance: Health Promotion/Disease Prevention**

CHAPTER 6: COMMUNICABLE DISEASES, DISASTERS, AND BIOTERRORISM

NCLEX® CONNECTIONS

When reviewing the content in this chapter, keep in mind the relevant sections of the NCLEX® outline, in particular:

CLIENT NEEDS: SAFETY AND INFECTION CONTROL

Relevant topics/tasks include:
- Emergency Response Plan
  - Use clinical decision-making/critical thinking for emergency response plan.
- Handling Hazardous and Infectious Materials
  - Identify biohazardous, flammable and infectious materials.
- Standard Precautions/Transmission-Based Precautions/Surgical Asepsis
  - Understand communicable diseases and the modes of organism transmission.

CLIENT NEEDS: HEALTH PROMOTION AND MAINTENANCE

Relevant topics/tasks include:
- Health and Wellness
  - Assess the client's knowledge of immunization schedules and educate as needed.
- Health Promotion/Disease Prevention
  - Identify risk factors for disease/illness.

Chapter 6	Communicable Diseases, Disasters, and Bioterrorism

Overview

- Communicable disease has been a worldwide health problem for many years.

- Disaster planning and bioterrorism have become more visible to health care providers in recent years.

- The nurse can help the community by understanding communicable disease, bioterrorism, and disaster planning and providing education and intervening as needed.

Communicable Diseases

- Worldwide, infectious diseases are responsible for the deaths of millions each year.

- Most deaths are from pneumonia, diarrheal diseases, tuberculosis, malaria, measles, and HIV/AIDS.

- Populations at risk for communicable disease include:

  o Young children

  o Older adults

  o Immunosuppressed clients

  o Intravenous drug users

  o Health care workers

- Routine immunizations for people of various ages are recommended by the Centers for Disease Control and Prevention (CDC). Recommendations are according to ages and include schedules/guidelines for people ages 0 to 6, 7 to 18, and 19 and up. The CDC Web site (http://www.cdc.gov) provides a quality resource for the most current information regarding immunization guidelines.

- Modes of Transmission

  o Airborne (inhaled by a susceptible host)

    ▪ Measles

    ▪ Chickenpox

    ▪ Streptococcal infection

    ▪ Tuberculosis

    ▪ Pneumonia

- Influenza
  - Foodborne (bacterial, viral, parasitic infection of food)
    - Salmonellosis
    - Hepatitis A
    - Trichinosis
    - Escherichia coli (E. coli)
  - Waterborne (fecal contamination of water)
    - Cholera
    - Typhoid fever
    - Giardia lamblia
  - Vector-borne (via a carrier such as a mosquito or tick)
    - Lyme disease
    - Rocky Mountain spotted fever
    - Malaria
  - Direct contact (skin-to-skin contact with mucous membrane discharges)
    - Sexually transmitted diseases (HIV, gonorrhea, syphilis, genital herpes, hepatitis B, C, D)
    - Infectious mononucleosis
    - Impetigo, lice, scabies
- Portals of Entry and Exit
  - Portals of entry
    - Respiratory system
    - Gastrointestinal tract
    - Skin
    - Mucous membranes
  - Portals of exit
    - Respiratory system
    - Feces
    - Blood
    - Semen/vaginal secretions
    - Saliva
    - Skin

- Defense Mechanisms
  - Natural immunity (from the body's antigen antibody response)
  - Artificial immunity (through vaccination)
    - Active (vaccination with live, killed, toxoid)
    - Passive (from antitoxin or antibodies)
- Prevention and Control Measures for Communicable Diseases
  - Infectious disease surveillance
    - The community health nurse engages in infectious disease surveillance, which includes the systematic collection and analysis of data regarding infectious diseases.
    - The CDC uses a four-level biosafety system to guide individuals in the care of those with communicable disease.
    - State law mandates which communicable diseases are reported to the CDC, and these vary by state. Some diseases included in the National Notifiable Diseases Surveillance System are:
      - AIDS
      - Anthrax
      - Botulism
      - Cholera
      - Diphtheria
      - Encephalitis
      - Giardiasis
      - Gonorrhea
      - Hepatitis A-D
      - Influenza activity
      - Legionellosis/Legionnaires' disease
      - Leprosy
      - Lyme disease
      - Malaria
      - Meningococcal infections
      - Mumps
      - Pertussis
      - Poliomyelitis
      - Rabies
      - Rocky Mountain spotted fever

- ▢ Rubella
- ▢ Rubeola (measles)
- ▢ Salmonellosis
- ▢ Shigellosis
- ▢ Severe acute respiratory syndrome-associated Coronavirus disease (SARS-CoV)
- ▢ Syphilis
- ▢ Smallpox
- ▢ Tetanus
- ▢ Toxic shock syndrome
- ▢ Trichinosis
- ▢ Tuberculosis
- ▢ Typhoid fever
- ▢ Vancomycin-resistant Staphylococcus aureus (VRSA)
- ▢ Varicella (chickenpox)
- o Health care goals regarding the control of communicable diseases
  - ■ Reductions in:
    - ▢ Cases of vaccine-preventable disease among lower-income populations
    - ▢ Pneumococcal and meningococcal infections for high-risk clients such as older adults or college students
    - ▢ Tuberculosis for high risk groups such as homeless or older adults
    - ▢ Group B streptococcal disease in newborns
    - ▢ Antibiotics for ear infections in children to prevent resistance
  - ■ Increases in:
    - ▢ Number of tuberculosis patients who complete therapy
    - ▢ Number of travelers who receive recommended preventive services, particularly if traveling in a high-risk area
    - ▢ Vaccination coverage, particularly for high-risk populations
    - ▢ General safety levels for food production
    - ▢ Use of condoms for the prevention of sexually transmitted diseases
- o Immunization
  - ■ The community health nurse plays a major role in increasing immunization coverage.
  - ■ Immunizations are often administered in community health settings, such as public health departments.

Ⓖ

- The community health nurse often tracks immunization schedules of at-risk populations such as children, elderly, immunosuppressed, intravenous drug abusers and health care workers.

- The community health nurse must educate the community about the importance of immunizations.

- The community health nurse must stay up to date on current immunization schedule recommendations and appropriate precautions when administering immunizations.

  o Levels of prevention

PRIMARY PREVENTION	SECONDARY PREVENTION	TERTIARY PREVENTION
• Prevent the occurrence of infectious disease. • Educate the public regarding the need for immunizations, federal and state vaccination programs, and immunization laws such as the "no-shots, no school" legislation. • Counsel clients traveling to other countries about protection from infectious diseases. Refer clients to the health department for information about mandatory immunizations. • Educate the public regarding prevention of disease and ways to eliminate risk factors for exposure, such as hand hygiene, universal precautions, proper food handling and storage, and use of condoms.	• Increase early detection through screening and case finding. • Refer suspected cases of communicable disease for diagnostic confirmation and epidemiologic reporting. • Treat postexposure infections (hepatitis A, rabies). • Quarantine clients when necessary.	• Decrease complications and disabilities due to infectious diseases through treatment and rehabilitation. • Monitor treatment compliance, including directly observed therapy. • Prevent reinfection. Identify community resources.

Disasters

- A disaster is an event that causes human suffering and demands more resources than are available in the community. A disaster may be man-made or naturally occurring. A disaster can be major or catastrophic.

- Three Levels of Disaster Management

  o Disaster preparedness

    - This type of management includes preparedness for natural or man-made disasters.

- The Federal Response Plan is a government plan that includes the Federal Emergency Management Agency (FEMA), U.S. Public Health Service, and Centers for Disease Control and Prevention (CDC). The plan guides the coordination of efforts in response to a disaster.

- Predisaster planning should include identification and assessment of populations at risk.

  □ Populations at risk are those populations that have fewer resources or less of an ability to withstand and survive a disaster without physical harm.

  □ These populations tend to be physically isolated, disabled, or unable to access disaster services. Strategic emergency planning is necessary to prevent the loss of lives in susceptible populations.

- Disaster preparedness should include planning for the possibility of worldwide pandemics (WHO/HHS Pandemic Avian Influenza Plan of 2005). Individual disaster preparedness should include: an action plan with communication, evacuation route, and disaster kit.

- Setting up a communication protocol is an important part of disaster planning. The communication plan should provide for access to emergency agencies, such as the American Red Cross. This plan may be in-house, local, state-wide, or national, depending on the size of the disaster.

- Mass casualty drills are drills or mock disasters where personnel practice duties in a planned disaster scenario.

○ Disaster response

- Different agencies are responsible for different levels of disaster response. They include FEMA, the Office of Emergency Management (OEM), and the American Red Cross. At the local level, hospitals, emergency departments, public health departments, mental health workers, and rescue personnel are responsible and have separate disaster duties.

- Disaster management response includes an initial assessment of the span of the disaster. This includes:

  □ How many people are affected?

  □ How many are injured or dead?

  □ How much fresh water and food is available?

  □ What are the areas of risk or sanitation problems?

- Nursing roles during a disaster response include triaging victims with serious versus minor injuries, prioritizing care of victims, and transferring those requiring immediate attention to medical facilities.

  □ Triage includes freeing acute care beds by determining which clients can be discharged (those who are hospitalized for diagnosis or observation).

  □ Other roles include giving tetanus shots, first aid, and medical attention to victims.

  □ Shelter nursing is a unique role of the nurse that can extend into the recovery phase of the disaster.

- ○ Disaster recovery

    - ▪ Recovery is the length of time that it takes involved agencies to restore the economic and civil life of the community. At an individual level, it is the time it takes an individual to become a functioning person within a community after a disaster.

    - ▪ Plague and sanitation controls are important aspects of disaster recovery. In the Pakistani-Indian earthquake of 2005, tetanus became epidemic due to the lack of vaccines, the remoteness of villages, the isolation of populations, and the number of infected wounds.

    - ▪ Posttraumatic stress disorder (PTSD) and delayed stress reactions (DSR) are common during the aftermath of disasters and may affect both caregivers and victims.

    - ▪ Phases of emotional reaction during a disaster

        - □ Heroic – Occurs at the time of the disaster. Intense excitement and concern for survival.

        - □ Honeymoon – Postdisaster period (two weeks to two months). Individuals feel support from government.

        - □ Disillusionment – lasts for several months to a year or more. Phase contains unexpected delays in receiving aid.

        - □ Reconstruction – Lasts several years and is the attempt to rebuild.

    - ▪ Nursing roles in disaster recovery include stress counseling, home health care, and reassessment of health care needs of the affected population.

- • Roles of Community Health Nurses in Disaster Management

    - ○ Participation in risk assessment includes asking the following questions:

        - ▪ What are the populations at risk within the community?

        - ▪ Have there been previous disasters, natural or man-made?

        - ▪ What size of an area or population is likely to be affected in a worst-case scenario?

        - ▪ What is the community disaster plan?

        - ▪ What kind of warning system is in place?

        - ▪ What types of disaster response teams (volunteers, nurses, health professionals, emergency medical technicians, firemen) are in place?

        - ▪ What kinds of resource facilities (hospitals, shelters, churches, food-storage facilities) are available in the event of a disaster?

        - ▪ What type of evacuation measures (boat, motor vehicle, train) will be needed?

        - ▪ What type of environmental dangers (chemical plants, sewage displacement) may be involved?

- o Participation in community disaster planning includes:
  - Developing a disaster response plan based on the most probable disaster threats.
  - Identifying the community disaster warning system and communication center, and learning how to access it.
  - Identifying the first responders in the community disaster plan.
  - Making a list of agencies that are available for the varying levels of disaster management, both locally and nationally.
  - Defining the nursing roles in first priority, second priority, and third priority triage.
  - Identifying the specific roles of personnel involved in disaster response and the chain of command.
  - Locating all equipment and supplies needed for disaster management, including hazmat suits, infectious control items, medical supplies, food, and potable water. Replenish these regularly.
  - Checking equipment (including evacuation vehicles) regularly to ensure proper operation.
  - Evaluating the efficiency, response time, and safety of disaster drills, mass casualty drills, and disaster plans.
- o Participation in community disaster response includes:
  - Participating in community disaster plans.
  - Activating the disaster management plan.
  - Performing triage and directing disaster victims, evacuation, quarantine, and management of shelters.
  - Assessing disaster victims and caretakers for posttraumatic stress disorder (PTSD) or delayed stress reactions, and giving them psychological treatment after the disaster.
- o Participation in evaluation of community disaster response includes:
  - Evaluating the area, effect, and level of the disaster.
  - Creating ongoing assessment and surveillance reports.
  - Evaluating the efficiency of the disaster response teams.
  - Estimating the length of time for recovery of community services, such as electricity and running potable water.

Bioterrorism

- Agents of Bioterrorism
  - o Category A biological agents are the highest priority agents, posing a risk to national security because they are easily transmitted and have high mortality rates.
    - Examples include smallpox (variola), botulism toxin, anthrax, tularemia, hemorrhagic viral fevers, and plague.

- Category B biological agents are the second highest priority because they are moderately easy to disseminate and have moderate morbidity rates and low mortality rates.
  - Examples include typhus and cholera.
- Category C biological agents are the third highest priority, comprising emerging pathogens that can be engineered for mass dissemination because they are easy to produce, and/or have a potential for high morbidity and mortality rates.
  - Examples include Hantavirus.

INCIDENT	SIGNS AND SYMPTOMS	TREATMENT/PREVENTION
Inhalational anthrax	• Sore throat • Fever • Muscle aches • Severe dyspnea • Meningitis • Shock	• IV ciprofloxacin (Cipro)
Botulism	• Difficulty swallowing • Progressive weakness • Nausea, vomiting, abdominal cramps • Difficulty breathing	• Airway management • Antitoxin • Elimination of toxin
Smallpox	• High fever • Fatigue • Severe headache • Rash (begins on face and tongue, quickly spreading to the arms and legs, then hands and feet, within 24 hr) that turns to pus-filled lesions • Vomiting • Delirium • Excessive bleeding	• Treatment – No cure • Supportive care – Hydration, pain medication, antipyretics • Prevention – Vaccine (provides 10-year immunity)
Ebola	• Sore throat • Headache • High temperature • Nausea, vomiting, diarrhea • Internal and external bleeding • Shock	• Treatment – No cure • Supportive care – Minimization of invasive procedures • Prevention – Avoidance of contaminated items • Vaccine – In testing phase. None currently available.

- Delivery Mechanisms for Biological Agents
  - Direct contact (subcutaneous anthrax)
  - Simple dispersal device (airborne, nuclear)
  - Water and food contamination
  - Droplet or blood contact

- Role of the Community Health Nurse

  o Participate in planning and preparation for immediate response to a bioterrorist event.

  o Identify potential biological agents for bioterrorism.

  o Survey for and report bioterrorism activity (usually to the local health department).

  o Promptly participate in measures to contain and control the spread of infections resulting from bioterrorist activity.

- Assessment of Bioterrorism Threat

  o Is the population at risk for sudden high disease rates?

  o Is the vector that normally carries a specific disease available in the geographical area affected?

  o Is there a potential delivery system within the community?

- Recognition of a Bioterrorism Event

  o Is there a rapidly increasing disease incidence in a normally healthy population?

  o Is a disease occurring that is unusual for the area?

  o Is an endemic occurring at an unusual time? For example, is there an outbreak of influenza in the summer?

  o Are there large numbers of people dying rapidly with similar presenting symptoms?

  o Are there any individuals presenting with unusual symptoms?

  o Are there unusual numbers of dead or dying animals, unusual liquids/vapors/odors?

PRIMARY PREVENTION	SECONDARY PREVENTION	TERTIARY PREVENTION

• Preparation with bioterrorism drills, vaccines, and antibiotics for exposure prophylaxis
• Bioterrorism planning
  ○ Design a bioterrorist response plan using the most probable biological agent in the local area.
  ○ Assess and locate the local facilities that have Level I, Level II, Level III, and Level IV biosafety gear.
  ○ Identify the chain of command for reporting bioterrorist attacks.
  ○ Define the nursing roles in the event of a bioterrorist attack.
  ○ Set up protocols for different biosafety levels of infection control and containment.
	• Early recognition
	• Activation of bioterrorism response plan in response to a bioterrorist event
	• Immediate implementation of infection control and containment measures, including decontamination, environmental disinfection, protective equipment, community education/ notification, and quarantines
	• Screening the population for exposure, assessing rates of infection, and administering vaccines as available
	• Assisting with and educating the population regarding symptom identification and management (immunoglobulin, antiviral, antitoxins, and antibiotic therapy, depending on the agent)
	• Monitoring mortality and morbidity
		• Rehabilitation of survivors
		• Monitoring medication regimens and referrals
		• Evaluating the effectiveness and timeliness of the bioterrorism plan

CHAPTER 6: COMMUNICABLE DISEASES, DISASTERS, AND BIOTERRORISM

Ⓐ Application Exercises

1. A young adult has been diagnosed with a communicable disease that is airborne. Which of the following has this young adult likely contracted?

    A. Cholera

    B. Malaria

    C. Influenza

    D. Salmonellosis

2. A community health nurse is discussing the portals of entry and exit. Which of the following is a portal of entry? (Select all that apply.)

    _____ Blood

    _____ Skin

    _____ GI tract

    _____ Saliva

    _____ Mucous membranes

3. A community health nurse is teaching primary prevention measures to a group of individuals at the community health center. Which of the following is an example of primary prevention?

    A. Educating on the use of condoms

    B. Treating sexually transmitted diseases

    C. Prevent reinfection

    D. Referring suspected cases of sexually transmitted diseases

4. The disaster management plan has three levels. Which of the following is included in the preparedness level?

    A. Identification of risk populations

    B. Transferring of individuals

    C. Prioritizing care of individuals

    D. Home health care interventions

5. A community health nurse is educating the public on the agents of bioterrorism. Which of the following is a Category A biological agent? (Select all that apply.)

    _____ Hantavirus

    _____ Typhus

    _____ Plague

    _____ Tularemia

    _____ Botulism

6. A community health nurse is caring for a client who is receiving ciprofloxacin (Cipro) intermittent IV bolus for disease that he has contracted. Which of the following has the client likely contracted?

    A. Botulism

    B. Ebola

    C. Smallpox

    D. Anthrax

7. A community health nurse is a first responder to a bombing incident and is assigned to the triage area. Which of the following victims with life-threatening injuries should be given the highest priority?

    A. The most seriously injured victims

    B. Victims with the highest probability for survival

    C. Victims needing immediate transportation to a trauma center

    D. Victims at the highest risk for systemic complications

8. In the event of a smallpox threat, would individuals who were vaccinated against smallpox prior to 1972 (when smallpox was eradicated in the United States) need to be vaccinated? Why or why not?

_____

Scenario: A community health nurse is working in a county clinic where five cases of avian influenza virus have been confirmed (positive blood samples). The public health department has been notified.

_____

9. What should be the community health nurse's next action?

10. What phase of disaster management is this?

CHAPTER 6: COMMUNICABLE DISEASES, DISASTERS, AND BIOTERRORISM

 Application Exercises Answer Key

1. A young adult has been diagnosed with a communicable disease that is airborne. Which of the following has this young adult likely contracted?

    A. Cholera

    B. Malaria

    C. Influenza

    D. Salmonellosis

Influenza transmission is airborne (inhalation by a susceptible host). Malaria is vector-borne. Cholera is waterborne. Salmonellosis is foodborne.

 NCLEX® Connection: Safety and Infection Control, Standard Precautions/Transmission-Based Precautions/Surgical Asepsis

2. A community health nurse is discussing the portals of entry and exit. Which of the following is a portal of entry? (Select all that apply.)

    _____ Blood

    __X__ **Skin**

    __X__ **GI tract**

    _____ Saliva

    __X__ **Mucous membranes**

Portals of entry are defined as an area in which an infectious agent can enter the body. Skin is the No. 1 protective barrier but is also an entry for infectious agents. The GI tract and mucous membranes also are areas in which the infectious agents may enter. Blood and saliva are portals of exit for infectious agents.

 NCLEX® Connection: Safety and Infection Control, Standard Precautions/Transmission-Based Precautions/Surgical Asepsis

3. A community health nurse is teaching primary prevention measures to a group of individuals at the community health center. Which of the following is an example of primary prevention?

    A. Educating on the use of condoms

    B. Treating sexually transmitted diseases

    C. Preventing reinfection

    D. Referring suspected cases of sexually transmitted diseases

Primary prevention is aimed at the avoidance of disease. Educating on the use of condoms will assist in the avoidance of sexually transmitted diseases. Treating sexually transmitted diseases and referring suspected cases of sexually transmitted diseases are secondary levels of prevention. Preventing reinfection is tertiary prevention.

NCLEX® Connection: Health Promotion and Maintenance, Health Promotion/Disease Prevention

4. The disaster management plan has three levels. Which of the following is included in the preparedness level?

A. Identification of risk populations

B. Transferring of individuals

C. Prioritizing care of individuals

D. Home health care interventions

Identification of risk populations is conducted in the preparedness stage. Identifying those individuals will allow the nurse to make arrangements to prevent the loss of life. Transferring of individuals and prioritizing care of individuals are considered part of the response stage. Home health care interventions are part of the recovery stage.

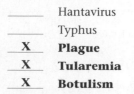 **NCLEX® Connection: Safety and Infection Control, Emergency Response Plan**

5. A community health nurse is educating the public on the agents of bioterrorism. Which of the following is a Category A biological agent? (Select all that apply.)

_____	Hantavirus
_____	Typhus
X	**Plague**
X	**Tularemia**
X	**Botulism**

Plague, tularemia and botulism are all category A biological agents. Hantavirus is category C and Typhus is category B.

NCLEX® Connection: Safety and Infection Control, Emergency Response Plan

6. A community health nurse is caring for a client who is receiving ciprofloxacin (Cipro) intermittent IV bolus for a disease that he has contracted. Which of the following has the client likely contracted?

A. Botulism

B. Ebola

C. Smallpox

D. Anthrax

Treatment for Anthrax is ciprofloxacin IV. Ciprofloxacin IV is not a treatment for botulism, which is treated with antitoxin. Smallpox and Ebola are treated with supportive care.

 NCLEX® Connection: Safety and Infection Control, Standard Precautions/Transmission-Based Precautions/Surgical Asepsis

7. A community health nurse is a first responder to a bombing incident and is assigned to the triage area. Which of the following victims with life-threatening injuries should be given the highest priority?

    A. The most seriously injured victims

    B. Victims with the highest probability for survival

    C. Victims needing immediate transportation to a trauma center

    D. Victims at the highest risk for systemic complications

In situations in which health resources are limited, a client's likelihood of survival must be the determinant of priority assignment. Community health nurses may be required to assist in deciding which clients to treat based on an assessment of each client's likelihood of survival with intervention. In these circumstances, priority is given to clients who have a reasonable chance of survival with prompt intervention. Clients who have a limited likelihood of survival even with intense intervention are assigned the lowest priority.

 NCLEX® Connection: Safety and Infection Control, Emergency Response Plan

8. In the event of a smallpox threat, would individuals who were vaccinated against smallpox prior to 1972 (when smallpox was eradicated in the United States) need to be vaccinated? Why or why not?

Yes: The smallpox vaccination provides only 10 years of immunity.

 NCLEX® Connection: Standard Precautions/Transmission-Based Precautions/Surgical Asepsis

---

Scenario: A community health nurse is working in a county clinic where five cases of avian influenza virus have been confirmed (positive blood samples). The public health department has been notified.

---

9. What should be the community health nurse's next action?

Priority should be given to containing the initial outbreak of a potential pandemic. Appropriate actions prior to the arrival of the public health department officials include initiating a quarantine of those inside the clinic (including staff) and closure of the clinic.

When public health department officials arrive, they will take blood samples for avian influenza DNA testing from the staff. A reportable communicable disease form needs to be completed for each of the confirmed cases. The public health department may involve the law enforcement agency to quarantine others as needed.

 NCLEX® Connection: Safety and Infection Control: Emergency Response Plan

10. What phase of disaster management is this?

This is the disaster response phase. This phase involves activation of the disaster management plan, triage and management of disaster victims, evacuation, quarantine, and management of shelters as needed depending upon the level of disaster.

 NCLEX® Connection: Safety and Infection Control: Emergency Response Plan

CHAPTER 7: CONTINUITY OF CARE

- Referrals, Discharge Planning, and Case Management
- Technology and Community Nursing
- Health Care With Faith-Based Organizations
- Partnerships in the Workplace
- Partnerships With Legislative Bodies

NCLEX® CONNECTIONS

When reviewing the content in this chapter, keep in mind the relevant sections of the NCLEX® outline, in particular:

CLIENT NEEDS: MANAGEMENT OF CARE

Relevant topics/tasks include:
- Case Management
  - Explore resources available to assist the client in achieving or maintaining independence.
- Collaboration with Interdisciplinary Team
  - Identify significant information to report to other disciplines.
- Concepts of Management
  - Act as a liaison between the client and others.
- Referrals
  - Identify community resources for the client.

Chapter 7   Continuity of Care

Overview

- Community health nurses play a large role in maintaining continuity of care for clients as they transition from inpatient to outpatient settings.

- Community health nurses use technology to maintain continuity of care.

- Community partnerships are essential to improving and maintaining healthy communities.

- Partnerships may be developed among individuals, families, community-based agencies, and/or citizen groups. Effective partners share similar goals and work together to achieve those goals.

EXAMPLES OF PARTNERING ENTITIES	GENERAL ISSUES PARTNERS MIGHT ADDRESS
• Individuals • Families • Community-based agencies • Civic organizations • Citizen groups • Educational settings • Political offices • Employment bureaus	• Information management • Cultural values • Health care system improvement • Physical environment

- Community health nurses should facilitate the development of partnerships within the community. These partnerships are important in the attainment of jointly desired health outcomes.

- Groups partnering to elicit needed change in the community are more powerful than a nurse working independently with an individual.

REFERRALS, DISCHARGE PLANNING, AND CASE MANAGEMENT

Overview

- A continuum of care assists in coordinating and providing individualized health care services, without disruption.

- Community health nurses facilitate continuity of care through case management services. These services include focused supervision for individualized care, follow-up, and referrals to appropriate resources.

- The establishment of an ongoing relationship between an individual and a health care provider leads to improved health outcomes.

Consultations

- A consultant is a professional who provides expert advice in a particular area. A consultation is requested to help determine what treatment/services the client requires.

- Consultants offer clients specialized knowledge or services (a cardiologist for a client who had a myocardial infarction, a psychiatrist for a client whose risk for suicide needs to be assessed).

- The nurse's role with regard to consultations is to:

    o Initiate the necessary consults or notify the primary care provider of the client's needs so the consult can be initiated.

    o Provide the consultant with all pertinent information about the problem (information from the client/family, the client's medical records).

    o Incorporate the consultant's recommendations into the client's plan of care.

    o Facilitate coordination of the consultant's recommendations with other health care providers' recommendations to protect the client from conflicting and potentially dangerous orders.

Referrals

- Referrals for individuals in acute care settings are typically based on the medical diagnosis, or other relevant clinical information. Resources assist in restoring, maintaining, or promoting health.

- The nurse assists in linking the client with community resources, and must have knowledge of individuals and organizations that can serve as resources.

- The nurse educates clients about community resources and self-care measures.

HEALTH CARE SERVICES	SUPPORT SERVICES
• Physicians • Acute-care settings • Primary care sites • Health departments • Long-term facilities • Homecare services • Rehabilitation services • Physical therapy services • Occupational therapy services • Specialty service agencies • Pharmacies	• Psychological services • Churches • Support groups • Life care planners • Medical equipment providers • Meal delivery services • Transportation services

- Steps in the Referral Process Include:
  - Engaging in a working relationship with the client
  - Establishing criteria for the referral
  - Exploring resources
  - Accepting the client's decision to use a given resource
  - Making the referral
  - Facilitating the referral
  - Evaluating the outcome
- Barriers to the Referral Process

CLIENT BARRIERS	RESOURCE BARRIERS
<ul><li>Lack of motivation</li><li>Inadequate information about community resources</li><li>Inadequate understanding of the need for referral</li><li>Accessibility needs</li><li>Priorities</li><li>Finances</li><li>Cultural factors</li></ul>	<ul><li>Attitudes of health care personnel</li><li>Costs of services</li><li>Physical accessibility of resources</li><li>Time limitations</li><li>Limited expertise working with culturally diverse populations</li></ul>

- Follow-up Considerations Include:
  - Monitoring to determine if the referral was completed.
  - Assessing whether referral outcomes were met.
  - Determining if the client was satisfied with the referral.

Discharge Planning

- Discharge planning is an essential component of the continuum of care, and is an on going assessment that anticipates the future needs of the client.

- Discharge planning requires ongoing communication between the client, nurse, physicians, family, and other health care providers. The goal of discharge planning is to enhance the well-being of the client by establishing appropriate options for meeting the health care needs of the client.

- The Joint Commission requires initiation of discharge planning at the time of admission to an acute-care facility.

Case Management

- Case management Nursing Includes:

  o Promoting interdisciplinary services and increased client/family involvement.

  o Decreasing cost by improving client outcomes.

  o Providing education to optimize health participation.

  o Advocating for services and client rights.

- Collaboration between clients, family, community resources, payer sources, and other health care professionals contributes to successful management of the client's health care needs.

- Case management nurses must possess excellent communication skills in order to facilitate communication among all parties involved. Being able to articulate the needs of the client to various parties can save time and unnecessary distress.

- Using the nursing process during case management will also help the client to obtain important services and to treat his condition.

APPLYING THE NURSING PROCESS DURING CASE MANAGEMENT	
Assessment	• Clarify the problem by evaluating physical needs, psychosocial issues, functional ability, and financial constraints.
Diagnosis	• Determine the cause and precipitating factors. • Identify applicable nursing diagnoses by using the above assessment.

Planning	• In conjunction with the client and family, determine:
	  o Possible outcomes for the client
	  o Advantages and disadvantages of possible outcomes
	  o What role each participant will play
	  o Impact on the client in each of the areas listed for the assessment

Intervention	• The case manager:
	  o Contacts service providers
	  o Provides referral information
	  o Coordinates all services to be provided
	  o Monitors the client to determine if services are still appropriate

Evaluation (continued monitoring)	• Monitor the care provided by the different agencies, comparing against:
	  o Original projected outcomes
	  o Physical needs
	  o Psychosocial needs
	  o Financial needs
	  o Client and family satisfaction

- The nurse provides a link between all facets of the health care experience. This means coordinating care between the primary care providers, nursing staff, physical and occupational therapists, rehabilitation facilities, and home health care.

- The case manager must be proactive for the client, balancing the impact of the illness against the cost of care. Increased knowledge and awareness of the disease process will decrease hospital stays because of early intervention.

- Use of appropriate community agencies will also contain costs, because the monitoring of clients leads to better disease management.

TECHNOLOGY AND COMMUNITY NURSING

Overview

- Technological advances have led to drastic changes in the delivery of health care. The availability of new technologies results in a disruption of old delivery methods, while simultaneously creating new opportunities.

- The expense of new technology should be considered as implemented in the care of patients. Technology has had an impact on increasing life expectancy, yet may also lead to instances of ethical dilemmas in some situations.

- Nurses must remain appraised of new technologies in order to deliver optimal care. The introduction of new technologies can have a significant impact on communities, thus impacting health outcomes.

Informatics and Telehealth

- Informatics is the combination of nursing science with information and communication technologies in the delivery of nursing care.

  o Computerized records, databases, and billing are commonly used within current the health care industry. Personal digital assistants (PDAs), geographic information systems, and the Internet all play a role in the delivery of health care.

  o Meetings can be held electronically; chat rooms and asynchronous discussions can be used as an alternative delivery method for health education, to facilitate support groups, or in staff or student orientations/training.

- Telehealth is the delivery of quality health care through the use of telecommunication technologies. Advances in communication technologies also allows for the delivery of education, and to increase awareness of health issues, through the use of telehealth.

  o Telehealth is particularly useful in rural areas. The ability to deliver specialized, skilled nursing through communications systems that transfers information easily between providers has greatly enhanced access to health care.

- o Telehealth technologies are increasingly being used as a component of home health services. In this setting, the nurse can provide care to clients at home, while working from a central location, such as an office or health care agency. With the use of telehealth, however, it is important to balance the use of these services with actual hands-on care. A combination of these services is needed for optimal client outcomes.

- o Physical, audio, and visual data can all be transmitted using telecommunication technologies.

  - Physical data that may be transmitted includes:
    - □ Blood pressure
    - □ Weight
    - □ Blood oxygenation
    - □ Blood glucose
    - □ Heart rate
    - □ Temperature
    - □ ECG results

  - Audio data that may be transmitted includes:
    - □ Voice conversation
    - □ Heart sounds
    - □ Lung sounds
    - □ Bowel sounds

  - Visual data that may be transmitted includes:
    - □ Images of wounds
    - □ Images of surgical incisions

HEALTH CARE WITH FAITH-BASED ORGANIZATIONS

Overview

- Faith-based organizations are comprised of communities within a variety of religious groups that emphasize spirituality as an important component of health and wellness. Most religions have practices that are important to health and healing, and many follow specific practices when caring for an ill or dying member.

- Members of faith communities represent the entire life span, and all family types. This offers nurses the opportunity to work with a diversified population within the same setting.

- Caring and spirituality are central among faith-based organizations.

  o CIRCLE Model of Spiritual Care

    - **C** aring

    - **I** ntuition

    - **R** espect for religious beliefs and practices

    - **C** aution

    - **L** istening

    - **E** motional support

Missionary Nurses

- Missionary nursing seeks to promote health and prevent disease by meeting spiritual, physical, and emotional needs of people across the globe. These nurses may be career missionaries, or may serve as short-term, volunteer, or part-time missionaries.

- Cultural and language barriers often impact the provision of care, and collaboration within the community is essential in meeting goals.

Parish Nurses

- Parish nurses promote the health and wellness of populations of faith communities. The population often includes church members and individuals and groups in the geographical community.

- Parish nurses work closely with pastoral care staff, professional health care members, and lay volunteers to provide a holistic approach to healing (body, mind, and spirit).

- Functions of the parish nurse include:

  o Personal health counseling (health-risk appraisals, spiritual assessments, support for numerous acute and chronic, actual and potential health problems)

  o Health education (available resources, classes, individual and group teaching)

  o Liaison between faith community and local resources

  o Facilitator support groups, change within the congregation, training volunteers)

  o Spiritual support (help identify spiritual strengths for coping)

PARTNERSHIPS IN THE WORKPLACE

Overview

- All work environments have associated risks. Health care in the workplace seeks to both promote health and prevent occupational illness and injury. Through improvement and maintenance of health, workplace expenditures are decreased by less sick time use, fewer workers compensation claims, and lessened use of group health coverage.

- Nurses function in numerous roles within workplace settings, and are challenged to provide cost-effective and high quality care. In this effort it is essential for the occupational health nurse to develop partnerships with workplace administration, industrial hygienists, safety specialists, occupational medicine physicians, human resource departments, union representatives, and health insurance agencies.

Occupational Health and Legislation

- The Occupational Safety and Health Act of 1970 established:

  - Occupational Health and Safety Administration (OSHA) – Develops and enforces workplace health regulations to protect the safety and health of workers.

  - National Advisory Committee on Occupational Safety (NIOSH) – Gathers and disseminates data on the incidence and prevalence of occupational illness and injury. This agency is also responsible for prevention education related to occupational injury and illness and determining hazards associated with new workplace technologies.

- Workers Compensation Acts – State-level legislation that regulates financial compensation to workers suffering from injuries or illness resulting from the workplace.

PARTNERSHIPS WITH LEGISLATIVE BODIES

Overview

- Decisions and actions made by legislative bodies can have profound impacts on health. Health policy specifically addresses health issues within public policy.

- To facilitate needed change, it is important for nurses to stay informed of current policy and laws that influence both the health of the community and nursing practice. Nurses should also advocate for policies that protect public health or offer solutions to community problems.

Nursing's Role in Health Policy

- Change Agents – Advocate for needed change at the local, state, or federal level.

- Lobbyists – Persuade or influence legislators. Lobbying may be implemented by an individual, or collectively through professional nursing associations.

- Coalitions – Facilitation of goal achievement through the collaboration of two or more groups.

- Public Office – Serving society and advocating for change by influencing policy development through public service.

CHAPTER 7: CONTINUITY OF CARE

 Application Exercises

1. A client is being discharged from the hospital to a rehabilitation facility following a stroke. Following 28 days in the rehabilitation facility, the client is anticipated to be discharged home, but will still need ongoing physical therapy. Discuss how the continuum of care can enhance the client's care.

2. List three benefits of the ensuring the continuum of care.

Scenario: A case manager is assigned the case of a 12-year-old boy who has recently been diagnosed with diabetes mellitus. He is unreceptive to learning about his disease and does not want to learn to read the glucometer or to give his own insulin shots. Although he has received some education about diet, he still eats what he wants, when he wants, without regard for his physical condition or blood sugar.

3. What communication techniques and approach should the case manager employ?

4. List techniques to help the client take responsibility for his diabetes monitoring and treatment.

5. Which of the following should the case manager suggest to keep this child from feeling alone with regard to his diabetes?

    A. Attend a diabetic camp for preteens.

    B. Go to a diabetic support group of various ages.

    C. Encourage the school nurse to meet and talk with him about diabetes.

    D. Tell his parents to emphasize the need for him to socialize.

CHAPTER 7: CONTINUITY OF CARE

 Application Exercises Answer Key

1. A client is being discharged from the hospital to a rehabilitation facility following a stroke. Following 28 days in the rehabilitation facility, the client is anticipated to be discharged home, but will still need ongoing physical therapy. Discuss how the continuum of care can enhance the client's care.

Through discharge planning the transition between the hospital and rehabilitation facility can be coordinated and implemented smoothly. This coordination would include planning and discussions amongst the client, family, each health care agency, and insurance or payers. Discharge from the rehabilitation facility would continue to include the client, family, agency, and payers; however referrals to a home health provider for continuation of physical therapy will likely be needed. Planning for needed assistive devices through a durable medical equipment company will assist the client to transition to life at home. Additionally, community referrals in the form of meal delivery, support groups, or care-giver support for the family might be needed. Ultimately, it is important to assess the individual needs of each client and family in order to coordinate needed care and help the client achieve the highest level of functioning possible.

 NCLEX® Connection: Management of Care, Continuity of Care

2. List three benefits of the ensuring the continuum of care.

1. Assists in cost containment

2. Ensures client health needs are met to enhance health outcomes

3. Enables nurses to gain knowledge of community members and groups that share similar goals. Knowledge of community resources assists not only in client care, but also in community-building through collaborative efforts.

 NCLEX® Connection: Management of Care, Continuity of Care

Scenario: A case manager is assigned the case of a 12-year-old boy who has recently been diagnosed with diabetes mellitus. He is unreceptive to learning about his disease and does not want to learn to read the glucometer or to give his own insulin shots. Although he has received some education about diet, he still eats what he wants, when he wants, without regard for his physical condition or blood sugar.

3. What communication techniques and approach should the case manager employ?

Try to reach the client at his level. Have him practice with the glucometer in a nonthreatening environment. Let him meet other people his age who have been successful in monitoring and treating their diabetes. Show him some Internet resources for preteens on diabetes.

 NCLEX® Connection: Management of Care, Case Management

4. List techniques to help the client take responsibility for his diabetes monitoring and treatment.

> Education provides power, and there is a need to empower this client. Make him the expert on diabetes by providing information in a fun and informative way. Check the Internet for Web sites where he can interact with other preteens who have diabetes and learn what they do to manage their diabetes. Get him involved in a preteen diabetic support group. Part of this client's regimen will need to include feeling that he belongs to a group.

 NCLEX® Connection: Management of Care, Case Management

5. Which of the following should the case manager suggest to keep this child from feeling alone with regard to his diabetes?

A. Attend a diabetic camp for preteens.

B. Go to a diabetic support group of various ages.

C. Encourage the school nurse to meet and talk with him about diabetes.

D. Tell his parents to emphasize the need for him to socialize.

> The more fun he has while learning, the more the client will learn. Diabetic camps that are geared for specific age groups teach clients how to manage their disease while still enjoying a "normal" life. That's important for clients in this (and any) age group. Attending a support group of various ages is not beneficial for a preteen because they interact best with individuals of the same age group. While the school nurse can provide information on diabetes, the preteen is more receptive to information presented in a "fun" way such as day camp. Having his parents tell him that socializing is important will not be beneficial.

 NCLEX® Connection: Management of Care, Case Management

References

Marquis, B.L., & Huston, C. J. (2009). *Leadership roles and management functions in nursing: Theory and application* (6th ed.). Philadelphia, PA: Lippincott Williams & Wilkins.

Nies, M., & McEwen, M. (2007). *Community/public health nursing: Concepts of care in evidence-based practice* (4th ed.). St. Louis, MO: Saunders.

Stanhope, M., & Lancaster, J. (2006). *Foundations of nursing in the community* (2nd ed.). St. Louis, MO: Mosby.